Women and Cancer

ISBN 0-918393-31-0

Published by

Harrington Park Press, Inc., 12 West 32 Street, New York, New York 10001.

EUROSPAN/Harrington, 3 Henrietta Street, London WC2E 8LU England.

Harrington Park Press, Inc., is a subsidiary of The Haworth Press, Inc., 12 West 32 Street, New York, New York 10001.

Women and Cancer was originally published in 1987 by The Haworth Press, Inc. It has also been published as *Women & Health*, Volume 11, Numbers 3/4, Fall/Winter 1986.

Cover design by Marshall Andrews.

Library of Congress Cataloging in Publication Data

Women and Cancer

Reprint. Originally published: New York: Haworth Press, c1986.
Includes Bibliographies.
1. Women—Diseases. 2. Cancer. 3. Cancer—Social aspects. 4. Cancer—Epidemiology. 5. Women—Tobacco use. I. Stellman, Steven D. [DNLM: 1. Neoplasms. 2. Women. QZ 200 W8715]
RC281.W65W64 1986 616'4'008042 86-26942
ISBN 0-918393-31-0

CONTENTS

EDITOR

JEANNE M. STELLMAN, PhD, *Associate Professor, School of Public Health and Executive Director, Women's Occupational Health Resource Center, Columbia University, New York, NY.* Dr. Stellman holds a doctorate in physical chemistry and is an associate professor in the School of Public Health at Columbia University, as well as Executive Director of its Women's Occupational Health Resource Center, which she founded in 1978. She is the author of several books including *Women's Work, Women's Health* (Pantheon, 1978), *Work is Dangerous to Your Health* with Susan Daum (Pantheon, 1973); and *Office Work Can Be Dangerous to Your Health,* with Mary Sue Henifin (Pantheon, 1983). She has written many scientific and popular articles and held a variety of advisory positions to government, labor, the women's movement and the scientific community, including chairing the March of Dimes Taskforce on Reproductive Hazards in the Workplace. She is currently co-editing an encyclopedia of occupational safety and health with Jacqueline Messite (Chapman-Hall).

BOOK REVIEW EDITOR

JANIS BARRY, PhD, *Assistant Professor, Division of Social Sciences, Fordham University, New York, NY.* Dr. Barry is an economist with a doctorate from the New School for Social Research. She has recently completed an extensive study on the relationship between economic compensation and women's employment in hazardous industries. She is an assistant professor in the Division of Social Sciences, Fordham University, New York, NY.

WOMEN'S HEALTH AND THE LAW EDITOR

MARY SUE HENIFIN, JD, MPH, *Consultant to the Women's Occupational Health Resource Center, Columbia University and Clerk to the Federal District Court, Newark, NJ.* Ms. Henifin holds a law degree from Rutgers University, a Masters in Public Health from Columbia and an undergraduate degree from Harvard. She is co-author, with Jeanne Stellman, of *Office Work Can Be Dangerous to Your Health* (Pantheon, 1983), editor of *Biological Women: The Convenient Myth* and *Women Look at Biology Looking at Women* (Schenckman 1979 and 1982). She is currently a clerk to Judge Debevoise, Federal District Court, and an active consultant to the Women's Occupational Health Resource Center, Columbia University.

HISTORICAL PERSPECTIVES ON WOMEN'S HEALTH EDITOR

DAVID ROSNER, PhD, *Associate Professor, Department of History, Baruch College, New York, NY.* Dr. Rosner is Associate Professor of History at Baruch College and the City University Graduate Center Doctoral Faculty. He received his PhD in the History of Science from Harvard and an MSPH from the University of Massachusetts. He is author and editor of four books including *A Once Charitable Enterprise, Hospitals and Health Care in Brooklyn and New York, 1885-1915* (Cambridge University Press, 1982); *Health Care in America,* (edited with Susan Reverby, Temple UP, 1979); *Dying for Work, Occupational Safety and Health in the United States,* (edited with Gerald Markowitz, forthcoming, Indiana); *Slaves of the Depression,* (with Gerald Markowitz, forthcoming, Cornell). He has served on the editorial board of Health PAC and on the APHA Medical Care Section Council.

FILM REVIEW EDITOR

CANDIDA PALTIEL, MFA, *Freelance film producer, New York, NY.* Ms. Paltiel holds a Masters in Fine Arts from Columbia University and is a freelance film producer. She is currently developing an educational module on the safe use of cancer chemotherapeutic agents in the workplace.

(continued on page xii)

Women and Cancer

Introduction

This collection of research papers, essays, and "thought-pieces" deals with the topic of cancer in women in both a scientific and social context. The papers cover the broad disciplines of epidemiology, screening, treatment, and ethics, as well as the narrower but extremely relevant area of tobacco usage.

One might at first wonder what is especially original about the individual topics covered here. Each has been treated before in its own corner of the cancer literature. Entire books can be found which cover in depth cancer epidemiology, screening, and treatment.

The thread which binds these papers together is not merely that they deal with cancer as it affects women—as individuals at risk, as patients, as caretakers for patients—but that the lessons to be learned from these studies can ultimately help us reduce the impact of cancer on our society, as well as on individuals of both sexes.

The papers have been organized in five sections: basic statistics, screening and early detection, implications of treatment and its aftermath, risks and benefits, and tobacco.

STATISTICS

Each of the three statistical papers provides important lessons and insights. Devesa lays out in stark figures the scope of the problem of cancer on a national basis: how many new cases arise each year, how many die, how many survive, and most importantly how these figures are changing. At once we are struck by the bleak figures on the seemingly unending increase in lung cancer, which tends to mask the much better news concerning improvement in survival from other types of cancer, and declines in stomach and cervical cancer rates.

Is there something "special" or "different" about cancer in women compared with men, apart from anatomical sites? For that matter, are there racial or ethnic differences in incidence, mortality, and survival, and if so why? The papers by Newell and Mills and by

Funch examine these rates by socio-economic status and ethnic group. They find that major differences indeed exist, which are in the main attributable to "lifestyle" differences in the broadest sense: differences in income, diet, smoking, and probably access to the health care system.

SCREENING AND EARLY DETECTION

One of the accepted dogmas of cancer education is that early detection of a cancer can lead to complete cure or at least increased survival. The three types of cancer in women which are most amenable to early detection are cervix, breast, and colon-rectum; an analogy for men exists only for the latter. Secondary prevention of cervical cancer through Pap smears is one of the triumphs of twentieth century medicine. Yet, Fisher and Page have discovered a weakness in the system: lack of systematic screening of high-risk women in an economically depressed area. Breast self-examination is another cheap yet effective screening method; most breast cancers are found by the woman herself. Hailey has measured compliance in a highly educated group (college women), and looked at reasons why some women do not practice this potentially life-saving technique.

Detection of colorectal cancer occurs mainly through gradual notice of often vague symptoms. As with many other cancers, delay in diagnosis and treatment can mean the difference between life and death. Marshall and Funch have studied whether men and women differ in the delay between recognizing and responding to symptoms, and furthermore whether physician diagnosis and treatment times differ.

TREATMENT

Practically all systemic cancers in our society are eventually treated in one way or another. Of the five papers on treatment and its aftermath, two deal with psychosocial aspects, but from nearly opposite perspectives. Penman and her colleagues have conducted a multi-institutional collaborative investigation of the impact of mastectomy on self-concept and other psychosocial outcomes. It has often been assumed that, compared with other forms of major surgery, mastectomy is unique in that, by depriving a woman of "femininity," it leaves her with reduced feminine self-image and produces other psychosocial disabilities. Penman finds very little evidence of this difference, and thus challenges a popular belief. This is a new and major finding. The study has been extremely well designed and carried out, with a convincing variety of control groups.

The second "post-treatment" paper, by Ulbricht, is just the opposite: it is a highly personal account of one woman's struggle to regain control of her life—and especially her speech—following surgical removal of her larynx. Besides being an inspiring, if understated, display of personal courage and strength, it also emphasizes the need for support groups for cancer patients (in this case, the International Association of Laryngectomees).

The two papers which follow also go in opposite directions, one dealing with the after-cancer life of the cured patient, the other with terminal care for the incurable. About half of all cancer patients can expect to live for at least five years past their diagnosis. Many can expect to return to a normal life, which includes earning a living. Feldman has surveyed former patients who have tried to return to work, as well as younger people looking for their first jobs. Some enlightened employers welcomed back their valued workers, making special allowances for reduced functionality. In too many cases, however, patients were let go, or quit following bad experiences with co-workers, or could not find new jobs because of their cancer history. Young women were often unable to obtain a first job because of their history. Health insurance was always a sore point, especially for the young. The entire question of job discrimination will receive more attention in the future as the number of former cancer patients working or seeking work grows. Feldman's paper is one of the few quantitative studies available; more are urgently needed.

Many cancer patients will unfortunately lose their battle. For them, the question is how to endure their final months or weeks with a minimum of pain, and how to die with dignity, for themselves and for their families. In a very brief time, as described by Hach and Wilson, the hospice movement has grown from a single institution to a network of several hundred, with a formal system of standards and Medicare certification. The hospice concept was begun and developed in the U.K. and U.S. by women; women also constitute the main caregivers, as nurses. Hospice has emerged as a highly humanistic oasis in an often impersonal medical care delivery system.

There is, regrettably, a seamy side of cancer treatment. It is perhaps inevitable that where large sums of money and fragile emotions are involved, opportunists take advantage of our incomplete ability to cure cancer by offering attractive but ineffective methods of their own. Brown has studied the strategems of cancer quacks and charlatans, and has summarized the methods used by purveyors of unproven methods of cancer treatment.

RISKS AND BENEFITS

Another pair of papers tackles the inevitability of trade-offs from two opposite extremes: that of the individual woman, and that of society as a whole. Barrett-Connor notes that the female hormone estrogen is widely prescribed to prevent bone mineral loss, but promotes cancer of the endometrium (uterine lining). Estrogen is also thought to prevent cardiovascular disease, but this protection is lost when progestin is added to counter the cancer risk. Uncertainties in this risk-benefit equation pose a challenge both to the woman and her doctor.

If this dilemma is faced by an individual woman, a different sort of dilemma is faced by society in balancing the individual's right to privacy with society's right to conduct research in order to set health policy for the benefit of all. Cancer studies in particular, as explained by Soskolne, pose a difficult problem. Our laws regarding disclosure of confidential data are becoming stricter, yet as knowledge grows, our need for new data, especially in treatment, is also growing. This inherent conflict poses ethical dilemmas which must be resolved.

TOBACCO

The final section of this volume is devoted to the greatest single acknowledged cause of cancer in women: tobacco. The subject of women and cigarette smoking has been treated in sufficient detail in the past, and a new recital of the dangers of smoking is not needed here; the information in the 1980 U.S. Surgeon-General's Report (The Health Consequences of Smoking for Women) is still fairly up to date and complete. Nevertheless, in view of the continued growth of the female lung cancer death rate, coupled with new developments in tobacco studies, a book on women and cancer would be badly deficient without some discussion of these topics.

One new and dismaying trend is the "feminization" of cigarette smoking in the U.S. While the smoking rate for men has been cut practically in half during the past twenty-five years, the rate in women has held steady or perhaps declined slightly. In recognition of this, or perhaps as a stimulus, the tobacco industry has targeted advertising at and developed brands specifically for women. Some of the new ads are portrayed in Ernster's article. Large advertising revenues may furthermore be partly responsible for the lack of anti-smoking information in otherwise "health-conscious" women's magazines.

The question "Is it harder for women to quit smoking than for men?" is taken up in a thought-piece by Orlandi. While cessation rates have differed in the past, the gap has closed in recent years. If there is a real difference, perhaps it means that different cessation strategies must be used for women. Such information is vital if we are to successfully reduce the prevalence of smoking in women.

Two final papers deal with smokeless tobacco and passive smoking. Even though use of snuff and chewing tobacco by women is a rather small problem nationally, Winn and Pickle point up the valuable lessons in epidemiology we have learned from studies of oral cancer in women in the rural South. Regrettably, this habit is increasing rapidly in men and boys, so that this lesson has much broader—and ominous—implications.

Finally, Papier and I review the evidence that breathing someone else's cigarette smoke can cause cancer in a non-smoker. Most studies have involved non-smoking women married to smokers, but there are also serious implications for the smokers' families, especially children. Furthermore, other health effects besides cancer can result from exposure to passive smoke. We also discuss some of the administrative remedies being undertaken, such as clean indoor air legislation and employers' no-smoking policies.

ABOUT THE AUTHORS

Even the statistically unsophisticated reader will notice a preponderance of women authors represented in this collection. While this was deliberate, it is by no means patronizing. The list of contributors includes many distinguished widely recognized leaders or future leaders in their respective fields. All in my opinion as editor have something important to say, and I consider myself fortunate, as well as honored, to have had the privilege of being the formal collector of these papers. (All papers were invited, except for two which had already been peer reviewed and accepted for publication at the time this volume was initially planned.)

ACKNOWLEDGMENTS

I would like especially to thank Lawrence Garfinkel, Vice President for Epidemiology and Statistics, and Director of Cancer Prevention of the American Cancer Society for making it possible for me to devote the necessary time to solicit, compile, and edit these papers. ACS Vice President Diane Fink was particularly helpful in suggesting topics and authors. I am grateful to Dr. Harold Freeman, Chairman of the ACS Subcommittee on Cancer Among the Economically Disadvantaged, for making it possible to publish Donna Funch's paper on socioeconomic status and survival. I wish I could thank by name the many anonymous reviewers who graciously consented to read and comment on these papers, but of course I can't. They provided needed expertise and filled in gaps in my own limited judgment and experience.

Finally, I am sincerely grateful to the Editor-in-Chief of *Women & Health* for her support and encouragement, as well as to my wife, Dr. Jeanne Mager Stellman, and rejoice in my good fortune that they are one and the same woman.

Steven D. Stellman

Cancer Mortality, Incidence, and Patient Survival Among American Women

Susan S. Devesa, PhD

ABSTRACT. Descriptive patterns of cancer among American women are presented utilizing national mortality statistics and data from several National Cancer Institute incidence surveys, the Connecticut Tumor Registry, the End Results Group Program, and the current Surveillance, Epidemiology, and End Results Program. From 1950 to 1980, deaths from cancer among women have become more numerous, but the overall age-adjusted mortality rates have not increased. Among white females, incidence and mortality rates for cancers of the stomach and cervix uteri have declined substantially during this time period, whereas lung cancer rates have increased dramatically. Improvements in survival rates are noteworthy for several types of cancer, including the leukemias, Hodgkin's disease, and the non-Hodgkin's lymphomas. There are substantial differences between the races and sexes in incidence rates by cancer site, and some differences in survival rates are also apparent. In the future, the numbers of women diagnosed with cancer will continue to increase as the larger cohorts of younger women age and as other causes of death continue to decline, with consequent increases in longevity. However, with the exception of lung cancer, large increases in rates for the common forms of cancer among women are not apparent.

This article provides an overview of the descriptive data regarding cancer among American women. Trends in mortality, inci-

---

Susan S. Devesa is with the Biostatistics Branch, Epidemiology and Biostatistics Program, National Cancer Institute, Bethesda, MD 20892.

This analysis would not have been possible without the efforts and contributions of many people, including the staffs of the surveys, registries, and SEER program, both around the country and at the National Cancer Institute; the programming assistance from the staff of ORI, in particular Mary Ann Read, Meg Seldin, and Ron Yeager; and Ruth Parsons of IMS. Critical review of the paper by Debra Silverman, Rochelle Curtis, and Joseph Fraumeni, Jr., is greatly appreciated. I am also grateful for typing of the manuscript by Rosie Strong and LaShonnah Tyson.

dence, and patient survival are presented by primary cancer site; and comparisons by race and sex are made using current incidence and survival rates. It is beyond the scope of this paper to summarize the risk factors that have been identified for these cancers or to correlate trends in the prevalence of these factors with the incidence or mortality trends. However, etiologic factors are discussed in the ensuing articles of this volume.

NUMBER OF DEATHS

Cancer is second only to heart disease as the most frequent cause of death among women in the United States; among those aged 35–54 years, it is the most frequent. During 1980, there were more than 190,000 deaths due to cancer among American women (National Center for Health Statistics [NCHS], 1985). Cancer is not one but many diseases, characterized by unrestricted cell proliferation and the potential for metastatic spread; if unchecked, it is usually fatal to the host. Table 1 presents the number of cancer deaths among American women during 1950 and 1980 (McKay, Hanson, & Miller, 1982; NCHS, 1985). During the 30 year period, the number of deaths due to all malignant neoplasms combined increased 84 percent from approximately 104,000 to 191,000. This trend reflects the increasing size of the U.S. population and shifts in the age distribution with a larger proportion of women in the older age groups, who are at higher risk of cancer. Total cancer mortality is also influenced by changes in the mortality rates for specific forms of cancer, changes in survival rates, and changes in the prevalence of risk factors influencing the incidence of the various malignancies.

The ten major sites of cancer among women are shown in Table 1 (listed according to rank in 1980). These cancers accounted for more than 75 percent of all cancer deaths among women at each point in time. The most frequent cause of cancer death in 1950 and 1980 was breast cancer; the numbers of deaths almost doubled during this period from about 19,000 to 36,000. In 1980, the next most frequent cause of cancer death was lung cancer, which increased more than 700 percent over the 30-year time period. As a percentage of all cancer deaths among women, deaths due to lung cancer rose from 3 to 15 percent. The numbers of deaths due to

Table 1.
Numbers of Cancer Deaths among Women in the United States: 1950, 1980

Cancer Site	YEAR 1950[a]	1980[b]
All Malignant Neoplasms	103,762	190,561
Breast	18,734 (1)	35,641 (1)
Lung	3,391 (9)	28,253 (2)
Colon and Rectum	17,207 (2)	28,189 (3)
Ovary	5,652 (6)	10,731 (4)
Pancreas	3,739 (8)	10,325 (5)
Lymphomas	3,130 (10)	10,223 (6)
Leukemias	3,787 (7)	7,367 (7)
Corpus Uteri	7,749 (5)	6,035 (8)
Stomach	8,978 (3)	5,858 (9)
Cervix Uteri	8,336 (4)	4,874 (10)
All Other Sites	23,239	43,065

Rank order indicated in parentheses.

[a]Source: McKay, Hanson, & Miller (1982).
[b]Source: NCHS (1983).

cancers of many other sites also increased. However, for several sites, the numbers of deaths have decreased, notably cancers of the cervix uteri, corpus uteri, and stomach.

The numbers of cancer deaths vary greatly by age group. During 1980, only six percent of all cancer deaths among women occurred among those less than age 45 years, whereas more than 60 percent occurred among women ages 65 and over (Table 2). The most frequent primary forms of cancer responsible for death also vary by age. Among females under age 25, the leukemias, brain and nervous system cancers, and lymphomas accounted for 60 percent of the cancer deaths. Breast cancer was the leading cause of death and lung cancer followed among women ages 25 to 64. The third most frequent site was the cervix among women ages 25 to 44, and the colon and rectum combined among those ages 45 to 64. Among women ages 65 and over, colorectal cancer surpassed both breast and lung cancers as the most frequent type. Colorectal, breast, and lung cancers accounted for 46 percent of the cancer deaths among women ages 65 and over.

Table 2.

Numbers[a] of Cancer Deaths among Women in the United States by Age Group, 1980.

	Age at Death (Years)			
	0-24	25-44	45-64	65+
Number of Cancer Deaths	1,910	9,556	62,035	117,060
% of Total Cancer Deaths	1.0	5.0	32.6	61.4
Most Frequent Cancer Cause of Death:				
1.	Leukemias (629)	Breast (2,956)	Breast (14,964)	Colorectal (21,101)
2.	Nervous System (326)	Lung (941)	Lung (12,258)	Breast (17,705)
3.	Lymphomas (183)	Cervix Uteri (811)	Colorectal (6,274)	Lung (15,044)
4.	Bones and Joints (150)	Leukemias (645)	Ovary (4,258)	Unknown Site (9,810)
5.	Endocrine Glands (107)	Colorectal (612)	Unknown Site (3,964)	Pancreas (7,574)

(Numbers of deaths shown in parentheses.)
[a]Source: NCHS (1983).

TRENDS IN MORTALITY RATES

The age-adjusted (1970 U. S. standard) mortality rates for all cancers combined decreased among white females by about nine percent from 1950 to 1977; among nonwhite females, the overall rates have remained fairly constant (McKay, Hanson, & Miller, 1982). In contrast, total cancer mortality rates increased 24 percent among white males and 71 percent among nonwhite males during the same period. However, notable differences in the trends by primary site were observed. Because mortality rates were not available for specific nonwhite racial groups in the past, the trends analysis has been restricted to white females.

In contrast to the increasing numbers of colorectal cancer deaths seen in Table 1, the average annual age-adjusted (1970 U.S. standard) mortality rates among white females have declined from the early 1950s to 1980 (Figure 1a). Stomach cancer mortality, which ranked third overall in 1950, has decreased dramatically over the entire time period, such that it now ranks in ninth position; the rate

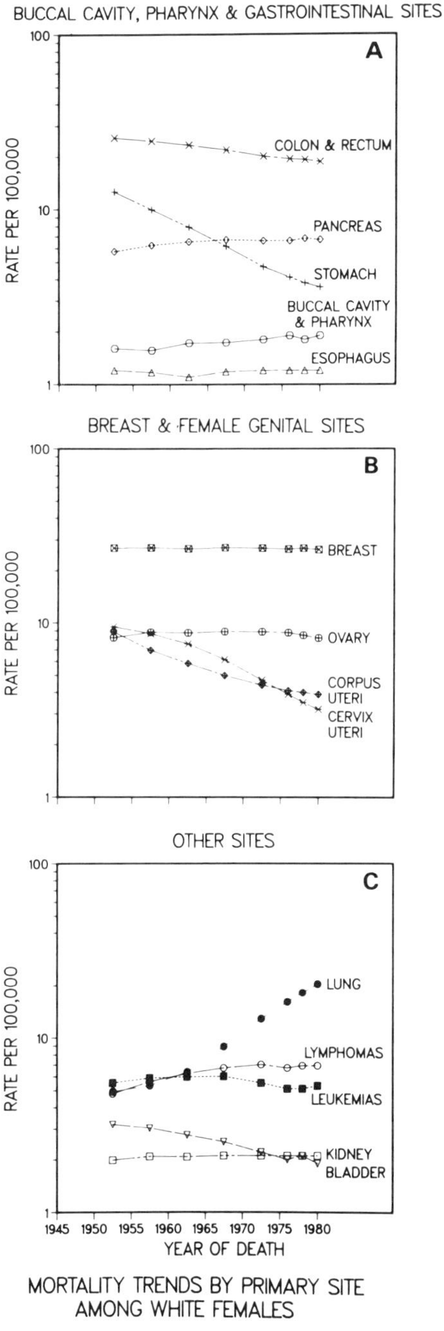

FIGURE 1.

Mortality trends by primary site among white females.

a. buccal cavity, pharynx, and gastrointestinal sites
b. breast and female genital sites
c. other sites

of decrease for stomach cancer is greater than that of any other cancer site. Pancreatic cancer mortality rates increased slightly during the early years, but they appear to have leveled off during recent years. Mortality rates for cancers of the buccal cavity and pharynx are quite low, and small increases over time are apparent. Esophageal cancer mortality is also rare among white females, and rates were fairly constant during the thirty years.

Among the reproductive sites, mortality rates for breast cancer among white females have remained remarkably stable over the 30-year period, and the rates for ovarian cancer also showed little change (Figure 1b). The rates for cancer of the cervix uteri declined substantially, at about four percent per year. Mortality rates for cancer of the corpus uteri (including uterus, not otherwise specified) also decreased, especially in the earlier years, but the overall change has been less than that seen for cervix cancer.

The rates for lung cancer, which was the ninth most frequent cause of cancer death among women in 1950, have increased more than those of any primary site (Figure 1c); the increases are more pronounced after the early 1960s. The lung cancer mortality rate surpassed that for colorectal cancer in the late 1970s, and it is projected that lung cancer deaths will surpass those due to breast cancer by the mid-1980s (U.S. Dept. of Health and Human Services, 1980). By 1983, the latest year for which data currently are available, this had already occurred among females in 15 states and among those ages 60–74 in the country as a whole. Mortality rates for the lymphomas (Hodgkin's disease, non-Hodgkin's lymphomas, and multiple myeloma) have leveled off during the 1970s following increases during the early years. Some decreases in the rates for the leukemias occurred during the late 1960s and early 1970s. Finally, bladder cancer mortality rates have declined at a fairly consistent rate over most of the 30-year time period, whereas the rates for kidney cancer have been remarkably constant.

INCIDENCE TRENDS

In contrast to mortality data, incidence data reflect numbers of newly diagnosed cases rather than numbers of deaths; however, such data are not routinely available for large portions of the country. The National Cancer Institute (NCI) has supported several surveys of cancer incidence in selected areas of the country: the first survey in 1937 (Dorn & Cutler, 1959), the second in 1947 (Dorn & Cutler, 1959), a special survey in Iowa in 1950 (Haenszel, Marcus, & Zimmerer, 1959), and the Third National Cancer Survey (TNCS) in 1969–71 (Cutler & Young, 1975). The original data from the first survey are not available, so the data presented in this report start with the late 1940s. Since 1973, the NCI-sponsored Surveillance, Epidemiology, and End Results (SEER) program has continuously gathered information on cancer incidence, mortality, and survival (Young, Percy, & Asire, 1981); the population-based registries participating in the SEER program cover more than 10% of the United States population. Since the same geographic areas have not been included in each of the surveys, direct comparisons of the published rates are not appropriate, except for selected registries. Of special interest is the tumor registry of Connecticut, which provides data for cases diagnosed since 1935 and is now a participant in the SEER program (Heston, Meigs, Kelly, & Flannery, 1985). Drawing on the above-mentioned sources, incidence trend data have been compiled for five geographic areas since the late 1940s: Atlanta, Connecticut, Detroit, Iowa, and San Francisco-Oakland (Devesa, Pollack, & Young, 1984). The populations in these five areas represented between 6 and 7% of the U.S. population at each point in time and, during the 1970s, represented about 72% of the SEER population. Comparison of the mortality rates in these five areas with those in the total U.S. revealed that, although the rates sometimes differed in absolute magnitude, there was quite good concordance in the secular trends by primary site (Devesa, Pollack, & Young, 1984). Due to differences over time in the reporting and the coding of some forms of cancer, it is not appropriate to estimate the long-term incidence trends for all cancers combined. Comparable data for trends analysis are available, however, for a number of individual sites.

For many cancer sites the trends in incidence differ somewhat from the trends in mortality. While mortality rates declined, the incidence of colorectal cancer showed little change among white females between the late 1940s and 1970, with small increases occurring since 1970 (Figure 2a). However, stomach cancer incidence rates have declined substantially, resembling the decreases observed in the mortality rates; over the time period shown, the rates dropped more than 70 percent, or about 4 percent per year. The incidence rates for pancreatic cancer increased from the 1940s to 1975 and then leveled off, whereas those for cancers of the buccal

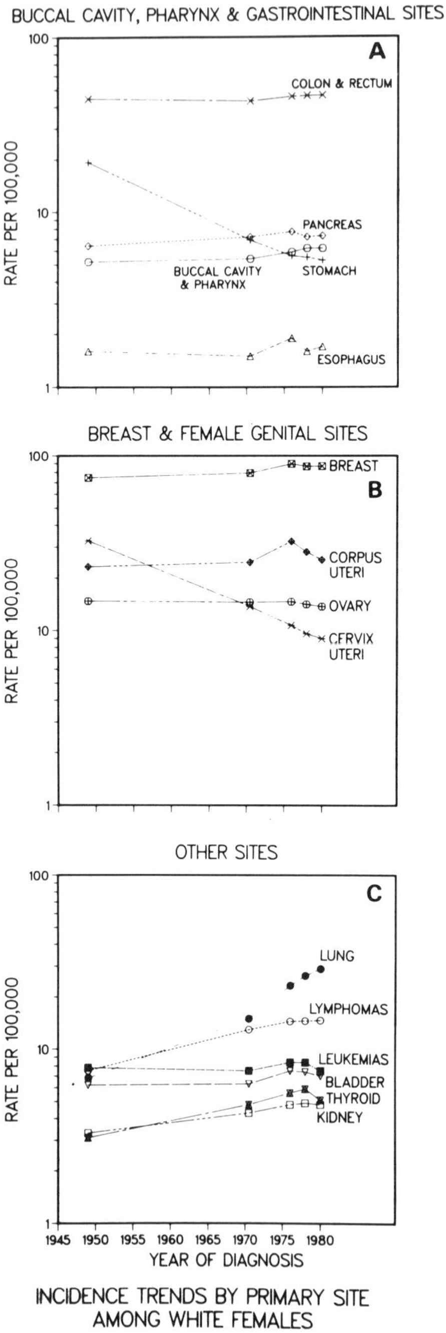

FIGURE 2.

Incidence trends by primary site among white females.
a. buccal cavity, pharynx, and gastrointestinal sites
b. breast and female genital sites
c. other sites

cavity and pharynx increased during the 1970s. The rates for esophageal cancer showed no consistent changes.

The incidence rate for breast cancer increased slightly from the late 1940s to 1970 (Figure 2b). During the mid-1970s, the increase became more pronounced, perhaps due to increased awareness of breast cancer and subsequent earlier diagnosis (Devesa, Pollack, & Young, 1984). The incidence of invasive cancer of the cervix uteri has declined dramatically, about 4 percent per year, in parallel with decreasing mortality. The rates are not shown for *in situ* carcinomas of the cervix uteri, which were seldom diagnosed during the late 1940s. By 1970, they were diagnosed twice as frequently as invasive cancers of the cervix; the *in situ*/invasive ratio increased to more than 3.0 during the late 1970s, primarily due to continued decreases in the rate of invasive cancer of the cervix. The decline in invasive cervical cancer incidence and mortality is at least partly due to the earlier diagnosis and treatment of lesions while *in situ* as well as to possible declines in the prevalence of risk factors, but the relative impacts of these factors are difficult to quantify. Cervical cancer rates shown in Figure 2b have not been adjusted to reflect the decreasing proportion of women at risk of developing cancer as a result of having a hysterectomy. When thusly adjusted, incidence rates show decreases of three rather than four percent per year. The trends for cancer of the corpus uteri, or total uterus excluding cervix, have been quite different. There was virtually no change in the incidence rate from the late 1940s to 1970; during the 1970s a sharp increase of more than 30 percent occurred, which has been followed by a decline. These trends follow closely the use of postmenopausal exogenous estrogens which has been shown to increase the risk of corpus uteri (endometrial) cancer (Marrett, Meigs, & Flannery, 1982; Austin & Roe, 1982). As with the mortality rates, age-adjusted incidence rates for ovarian cancer showed little change over the period for which data are available.

The incidence rates for lung cancer have increased more than those of any cancer site (Figure 2c), similar to the large increases in mortality. The incidence among white females increased from 6.8 to 28.9 per 100,000 per year, or more than 300 percent, over the 30-year period. Although the rates among females are considerably lower than those among males, the proportional increases are larger. Incidence rates for the lymphomas increased more than 90 percent during the early years, but they appeared to level off during the late 1970s. The lymphomas are a heterogeneous group consisting of

Hodgkin's disease, multiple myeloma, and other lymphomas. Despite the likelihood of different etiologies and time trends, there is a scarcity of long term incidence data for specific lymphoma types. A transient rise in the incidence rate for the leukemias, of which there are also a number of different types, is apparent during the mid-1970s. A similar pattern is seen for bladder cancer, whereas incidence rates for kidney cancer increased until the mid-1970s and remained stable thereafter. Finally, thyroid cancer incidence almost doubled from the late 1940s to the late 1970s. (Thyroid cancer was not included in Figure 1c because the mortality rates have been consistently less than one per 100,000 per year, due to favorable survival rates.) Incidence rates for skin melanomas increased during the 1970s (Horm, Asire, Young, & Pollack, 1984), not shown in the figure because rates for the late 1940s are not available.

CURRENT INCIDENCE RATES BY RACE AND SEX

As shown in Table 3, the overall age-adjusted incidence rate for cancers of all sites combined during 1978–81 was slightly higher among white compared to black females: 303 versus 290 per 100,000, respectively (Horm, Asire, Young, & Pollack, 1984). Racial differences in rates among females were minimal for the leukemias, kidney cancer, and lung cancer. However, rates were somewhat higher among white than black females for cancers of the breast, bladder, rectum, and ovary. Surpassing 50 percent were the higher rates among whites for cancers of the brain and other nervous system, thyroid, and corpus uteri, as well as the non-Hodgkin's lymphomas. Hodgkin's disease occurred more than twice as often among white compared to black females, and melanomas of the skin were extremely rare among blacks. However, a number of cancers occurred more frequently among black compared to white females, including slightly higher rates for cancers of the colon as well as the buccal cavity and pharynx. Pancreatic and stomach cancers occurred 50 percent more frequently among black females, and both cervix cancer and multiple myeloma were 130 percent higher than among white females. Finally, esophageal cancer was more than 3.5 times as common among black compared to white females.

There were also large differences in incidence rates between males and females (Table 3). Almost all cancers occurring in both

Table 3.

Incidence Rates[a] by Primary Site, Race and Sex: SEER Program, 1978-81

	Females		Males	
	Whites	Blacks	Whites	Blacks
All Cancer Sites[b]	303.2	290.3	391.9	487.9
Buccal Cavity and Pharynx	6.5	7.7	16.8	23.0
Esophagus	1.5	5.5	4.8	19.1
Stomach	5.2	8.3	11.9	21.3
Colon	31.7	36.6	39.0	39.9
Rectum	11.9	9.0	19.3	15.4
Liver	1.1	1.8	2.6	5.5
Gallbladder	1.8	1.2	0.9	0.9
Pancreas	7.3	11.1	10.9	16.8
Larynx	1.5	2.0	8.4	12.5
Lung and Bronchus	28.2	30.5	81.0	119.0
Melanoma of Skin	8.1	0.6	9.4	0.8
Breast	85.6	71.9	0.7	1.0
Cervix Uteri	8.8	20.2	-	-
Corpus Uteri	25.1	13.4	-	-
Ovary	13.6	9.5	-	-
Urinary Bladder	6.9	5.3	27.3	13.3
Kidney	4.4	4.5	10.0	9.2
Brain and Other Nervous System	5.0	3.0	7.1	4.4
Thyroid	5.3	3.1	2.1	1.2
Hodgkin's Disease	2.4	1.1	3.4	2.4
Non-Hodgkin's Lymphomas	9.2	4.9	12.2	9.0
Multiple Myeloma	2.9	6.7	4.1	9.6
Leukemias	7.5	7.3	13.0	10.9

[a] Average annual rates per 100,000 population, age-adjusted using the 1970 U.S. standard.
[b] Note: not all primary sites are shown individually.

Source: Horm, Asire, Young, & Pollack (1984) and additional tabulations.

sexes arose more often among males than females in both whites and blacks. Three notable exceptions are gallbladder, breast, and thyroid cancers. The rates for about one half the sites included in the table were less than twice as high among males than females of the same racial group. Rates among males were two to three times those among females for cancers of the kidney, stomach, liver, and buccal cavity and pharynx. Esophageal and laryngeal cancers were more than three times as common in males as females. Most of these sex ratios are similar among both blacks and whites. However, there are notable racial differences in the sex ratios for two sites: the male/female rate ratios for bladder cancer were 4.0 and 2.5 among whites and blacks, respectively, while the corresponding ratios for lung cancer were 2.9 and 3.9, respectively.

TRENDS IN SURVIVAL RATES

During the 1960s and early 1970s, the National Cancer Institute sponsored the End Results Program, which gathered information on the survival experience of cancer patients in a number of hospital registries and the population-based registry in Connecticut (Myers & Hankey, 1980). Since 1973, survival data have also been assembled as a part of the SEER program (Ries, Pollack, & Young, 1983; Young, Ries, & Pollack, 1984). Often used as a measure of survival after the diagnosis of cancer is the five-year relative survival rate, which is the ratio of the observed survival rate to the expected rate for persons from the general population who are similar with respect to age, race, sex, and calendar time. Table 4 presents five-year relative survival rates among white females by primary site for cases diagnosed during several time periods (Myers & Hankey, 1980; Ries, 1985). Consistently low survival rates are observed for patients with cancers of the pancreas, esophagus, liver, gallbladder, lung, or stomach; although some improvements are reported, five-year survival rates for these cancers are still less than 20 percent. Recent survival rates have been 75 percent or greater for patients with skin melanoma, Hodgkin's disease, and cancers of the thyroid, corpus uteri, or breast. Substantial variations in survival rates are apparent for the major subtypes of leukemia, and improvements have occurred over time, particularly for those with acute lymphocytic leukemia. Increases in survival rates are also noteworthy for Hodgkin's disease (from 48 to 76 percent) and for the non-Hodgkin's lymphomas (from 31 to 49 percent). More modest gains are apparent for many of the other sites; ovarian cancer has shown the least change over time. Although some of the reported improvements in survival may be partially due to changing diagnostic practices or medical definitions, which may artificially alter the survival rates (Feinstein, Sosin, & Wells, 1985), it is likely that both earlier diagnosis and improvements in therapy have each made substantial contributions.

CURRENT SURVIVAL RATES BY RACE AND SEX

Based on cases diagnosed during 1973–79 in the population-based SEER program (Young, Ries, & Pollack, 1984), striking differences between races and sexes in the five-year relative survival rates for all sites combined are apparent (Table 5). Overall survival rates are

Table 4.

Trends in Five-Year Relative Survival Rates (percent) among White Females by Primary Site.

Site	1960-63[a]	1970-73[a]	1973-75[b]	1976-81[b]
Buccal Cavity and Pharynx	NR	NR	NR	NR
Esophagus	6	4	7	5
Stomach	13	14	15	17
Colon	44	50	49	53
Rectum	41	48	49	50
Liver	3	6	7	5
Gallbladder	9	9	8	9
Pancreas	2	2	3	3
Larynx	46	56	71	62
Lung and Bronchus	11	14	15	15
Melanoma of Skin	68	75	81	85
Breast	63	68	74	75
Cervix Uteri	58	64	68	67
Corpus Uteri	73	81	89	86
Ovary	32	36	36	37
Urinary Bladder	53	60	71	71
Kidney	39	50	48	50
Brain & Other Nervous System	21	22	22	23
Thyroid	87	87	92	94
Hodgkin's Disease	48	69	69	76
Non-Hodgkin's Lymphomas	31	43	45	49
Multiple Myeloma	10	17	25	24
Leukemias (major forms):				
Acute Lymphocytic	3	29	37	55
Chronic Lymphocytic	46	59	69	70
Acute Granulocytic	0	2	5	8
Chronic Granulocytic	11	19	26	25

[a] Rates are based on data from a series of hospital registries and one population-based registry. Source: Myers & Hankey (1980).

[b] Rates are from the population-based SEER program and include patients diagnosed through 1981 and follow-up on all patients through 1982. Source: Ries (1985)

NR = not reported

higher among whites than blacks within each sex, and rates among females are higher than those among males within each race. These overall differences are to a large extent due to the race/sex differences in incidence rates for the various primary sites and to their associated variations in subsequent survival rates. When individual sites are considered, much less variation is apparent. Among females, survival rates among blacks are equal to or higher than those among

Table 5.
Five-Year Relative Survival Rates (percent) by Primary Site, Race, and Sex: SEER Program, 1973-79.

	Females		Males	
	Whites	Blacks	Whites	Blacks
All Sites Combined[a]	55	44	40	29
Buccal Cavity and Pharynx	NR	NR	NR	NR
Esophagus	6	5	4	2
Stomach	15	14	13	14
Colon	50	45	48	43
Rectum	48	41	46	32
Liver	6	8	2	NR
Gallbladder	7	10	9	16
Pancreas	3	4	3	2
Larynx	66	62	66	55
Lung and Bronchus	15	13	11	9
Melanoma of Skin	83	67	73	45
Breast	73	61	NR	NR
Cervix Uteri	67	62	-	-
Corpus Uteri	87	56	-	-
Ovary	36	38	-	-
Urinary Bladder	70	38	73	52
Kidney	48	58	49	46
Brain and Other Nervous System	23	31	19	15
Thyroid Gland	92	93	90	76
Hodgkin's Disease	72	68	67	70
Non-Hodgkin's Lymphomas	46	53	45	38
Multiple Myeloma	23	25	22	25
Leukemias	NR	NR	NR	NR

[a] Note: not all primary sites are shown individually.

NR = not reported

Source: Young, Ries, & Pollack (1984).

whites for liver, gallbladder, pancreatic, ovarian, kidney, brain, and thyroid cancers as well as for the non-Hodgkin's lymphomas and multiple myeloma. However, white females appear to have a survival advantage over black females for several cancers: bladder, corpus uteri, breast, and melanoma of the skin. When comparisons are made between the sexes, females have equal or higher survival rates than do males of the same race in the majority of instances. The only exceptions apparent are higher survival rates among males for gallbladder and urinary bladder cancer among both whites and blacks, kidney cancer among whites, and Hodgkin's disease among blacks; however, in most cases, the differences are minimal.

CONCLUSIONS

Although deaths from cancer among women have become more numerous, the overall age-adjusted mortality rates have not increased. Mortality rates for a number of the major sites have been fairly stable or have shown decreases. Large decreases in both the incidence and mortality rates for stomach and cervix cancer have occurred. Rates for lung cancer, however, have increased substantially, rising in incidence from ninth to third position. During the mid-1980s, lung cancer is expected to surpass all other types of cancer as a cause of death among American women. Dramatic changes over time in either incidence or mortality rates for breast cancer are not apparent, although it is the most common form of cancer diagnosed among women. Increases in the incidence rates for colorectal cancer, also a major primary site, are suggested only during the 1970s, while the mortality rates have declined consistently since the early 1950s. Improvements in cancer patient survival are noted for a number of cancers, particularly the leukemias, Hodgkin's disease, and non-Hodgkin's lymphomas. In the future, the numbers of women affected by cancer will continue to increase as the larger cohorts of younger women grow older and other causes of death continue to decline, with consequent increases in longevity. However, with the exception of lung cancer, large increases in rates for common forms of cancer among women are not apparent.

REFERENCES

Austin, D. F., & Roe, K. M. (1982). The decreasing incidence of endometrial cancer: Public health implications. *American Journal of Public Health, 72*, 65–68.

Cutler, S. J., & Young, J. L., Jr. (Eds.). (1975). Third National Cancer Survey: Incidence data. *National Cancer Institute Monograph 41* (Department of Health, Education, & Welfare Publication No. (National Institutes of Health) 75–787).

Devesa, S. S., Pollack, E. S., & Young, J. L., Jr. (1984). Assessing the validity of observed cancer incidence trends. *American Journal of Epidemiology, 119*, 274–291.

Dorn, H. F., & Cutler, S. J. (1959). Morbidity from cancer in the United States: Parts I and II. *Public Health Monograph 56* (Public Health Service Publication No. 590).

Feinstein, A. R., Sosin, D. M., & Wells, C. K. (1985). The Will Rogers phenomenon: Stage migration and new diagnostic techniques as a source of misleading statistics for survival in cancer. *New England Journal of Medicine, 312*, 1604–1608.

Haenszel, W., Marcus, S. C., & Zimmerer, E. G. (1959). Cancer morbidity in urban and rural Iowa. *Public Health Monograph 37* (Public Health Service Publication No. 462).

Heston, J., Meigs, J. W., Kelly, J., & Flannery, J. T. (1985). Forty-five years of cancer incidence in Connecticut: 1935–79. *National Cancer Institute Monograph 70* (National Institutes of Health Publ. No. 86-2652).

Horm, J. W., Asire, A. J., Young, J. L., Jr., & Pollack, E. S. (Eds.). (1984). *SEER Program: Cancer incidence and mortality in the United States, 1973–81*. Bethesda, MD: U. S. Department of Health and Human Services (National Institutes of Health Publication No. 85–1837).

Marrett, L. D., Meigs, J. W., & Flannery, J. T. (1982). Trends in the incidence of cancer of the corpus uteri in Connecticut, 1964–1979, in relation to consumption of exogenous estrogens. *American Journal of Epidemiology, 116*, 57–67.

McKay, F. W., Hanson, M. R., & Miller, R. W. (1982). Cancer mortality in the United States: 1950–1977. *National Cancer Institute Monograph 59* (National Institutes of Health Publication No. 82–2435).

Myers, M. H., & Hankey, B. F. (1980). *Cancer patient survival experience*. Bethesda, MD: U. S. Department of Health and Human Services (National Institutes of Health Publication No. 80–2148).

National Center of Health Statistics (1985). Computer magnetic tapes containing United States mortality data.

Ries, L. (1985). Unpublished data.

Ries, L. G., Pollack, E. S., & Young, J. L., Jr. (1983). Cancer patient survival: Surveillance, Epidemiology, and End Results Program, 1973–79. *Journal of the National Cancer Institute, 70*, 693–707.

U.S. Department of Health and Human Services. (1980). *The Health Consequences of Smoking for Women—A Report of the Surgeon General*. Rockville, MD: Office of Smoking and Health.

Young, J. L., Jr., Percy, C. L., & Asire, A. J. (Eds.). (1981). Surveillance, Epidemiology, and End Results Program: Incidence and mortality data, 1973–77. *National Cancer Institute Monograph 57* (National Institutes of Health Publication No. 81–2330).

Young, J. L., Jr., Ries, L. G., & Pollack, E. S. (1984). Cancer patient survival among ethnic groups in the United States. *Journal of the National Cancer Institute, 73*, 341–352.

Low Cancer Rates in Hispanic Women Related to Social and Economic Factors

Guy R. Newell, MD
Paul K. Mills, PhD

ABSTRACT. Differences in the occurrence of three common types of cancer among Hispanic compared to Anglo women are presented. These are cancers of the breast, colon, and lung, which together account for about half of all newly diagnosed cancers in the U.S. Differences occur in at least three different geographic areas, Texas, New Mexico, and Los Angeles. These cancer differences are presented in the light of some social and economic differences between Hispanic and Anglo women. Among them are several indicators of social class or economic development, fertility patterns, urban-rural differences, migration status and dietary habits resulting in different nutritional status between the two groups. Although a dietary hypothesis is attractive to explain the differences in breast and colon cancers, it is by no means proved. The magnitude of the differences in these cancers, coupled with their frequency of occurrence in the population, make them important sources for future study. The differences strongly suggest the existence of protective factors associated with ethnic-related life styles of Hispanic women.

INTRODUCTION

Spanish Americans or Hispanics are defined as persons of Mexican, Puerto Rican, Cuban, Central or South American or other Spanish culture or origin regardless of race.[1] There are three major subgroups of Spanish-Americans: Mexican-Americans, Puerto Ricans, and Cubans. The first subgroup resides mainly in California, Arizona, New Mexico and Texas; Puerto Ricans outside of

---

Guy R. Newell and Paul K. Mills are with the Department of Cancer Prevention, The University of Texas System Cancer Center, M.D. Anderson Hospital and Tumor Institute, 6723 Bertner Avenue, Houston, TX 77030.

Puerto Rico live predominantly in New York, Boston, Chicago, and Washington, D.C.; Cubans are concentrated in Miami.

Most descriptions of cancer differences have focused on populations or individuals at greater risk for certain types of cancer than other populations or individuals. This is important because such focus may suggest possible environmental or life style factors which may contribute to the cause(s) of the excess cancers. Spanish American women are known to experience more cancers of the gallbladder, bone, cervix, liver, nasal sinuses, and stomach than their Anglo American counterparts.[2] Less well recognized and investigated is that Hispanic women experience appreciably less of the most commonly occurring cancers, namely breast,[3] colon,[4] and lung,[5] than do their Anglo counterparts. This difference is also of considerable importance since it suggests there may be elements of personal environment or life style practices among these women which may protect them against developing these common cancers.

This discussion will focus on these variations in cancer occurrence between Anglo and Hispanic women with an attempt to explain some of them, although the reasons for all differences are not known. Particular attention will be focused on nutrition, fertility, socioeconomic status, urban or rural living patterns, smoking habits, and other possible factors.

SOURCES OF DATA

Sources of data pertaining to Hispanic groups in this country are relatively sparse and not uniform. Information on socioeconomic status and related factors are available from U.S. statistical reports,[6] and nutritional information was provided by a recent review.[7] Cancer incidence data were available for three geographic areas in the U.S. (Table 1).

All patients with cancer who resided in 56 Texas counties from January 1944 through December 1966 were ascertained.[8] Annual (1944–1966) and average annual (1962–66, 1949–1966, 1944–1966) age-specific and age-adjusted incidence rates per 100,000 were calculated. Three sets of rates were calculated based on three standard populations—U.S. 1950, 1960, and 1970. Spanish surnames were determined from a list of 6,000 Spanish surnames prepared by the U.S. Immigration and Naturalization Service.

The New Mexico tumor registry was established in 1969 and

Table 1. Characteristics of Areas Providing Cancer Incidence Data

Geographic Area	Years Covered	Population Base	Population Characteristics
Texas	1944-66	4.0 million	Anglos (53%)
			Hispanics (32%)
			Nonwhites (10%)
New Mexico	1969-76	1.0 million	Spanish or Mexican American (38%)
			American Indians (7%)
			Black (2%)
			Anglo (52%)
Los Angeles County	1972-76	7.5 million	Spanish ancestry, blacks, and Anglos

covers a population of approximately one million people, one-third of whom live in the state capital of Albuquerque. Thirty-eight percent of New Mexicans have Spanish or Mexican-American heritage, 7% are American Indians, 2% are black, and the remaining 52% are termed Anglo (of European descent, primarily from the British Isles). Surnames were divided into Spanish and nonSpanish categories using information from hospital charts and the detailed Spanish surname list from the 1970 U.S. census, in addition to a list of names developed specifically for New Mexico. New Mexico tumor registry data presented here include the years 1969 to 1976.

The Los Angeles County University of Southern California Cancer Surveillance Program is a rapid reporting system that collects from hospital pathology records all reported incidences of cancer in Los Angeles County.[9] Surnames were divided into Spanish and nonSpanish categories using the detailed Spanish-surname list from the 1970 U.S. census. The Los Angeles data include the years 1972 and 1976. In addition, Los Angeles has a large population of persons of oriental heritage, namely Chinese and Japanese.

RESULTS AND DISCUSSION

Ethnic and racial variation in the occurrence of different cancers led to the earliest suggestions that external environmental factors, rather than internal genetic or inherited predisposition, were responsible for the cause(s) of most human cancers.[10] Differences in all cancer sites among major ethnic groups residing in Los Angeles are shown in Table 2. Hispanic women experience more cancer than Chinese and Japanese women, but not as much as black and Anglo women. The remainder of this discussion will focus on cancer of major sites in Hispanic women compared with their Anglo counterparts. The term "Anglo" refers to Caucasian, nonHispanic women.

Among all cancer sites, those occurring in the female breast, large intestine, and lung comprise about 50% of all newly diagnosed cancers in this country. Thus, a reduction in cancers of these sites, as shown in Table 3, has great practical importance for public health aspects of cancer prevention. The data shown in Table 3 were collected by different groups, covering different time periods, and using different methods of ascertainment, reporting, etc. Thus, the differences are not necessarily comparable among the three geographic areas. In spite of the different methods, in each geographic area there are lower incidence rates in Hispanic women than in

Table 2. Incidence Rates per 100,000 for All Cancers by Ethnicity and Sex, 1972-1976

Ethnic Group	Women	Men
Chinese	181	258
Japanese	234	258
Hispanic	259	310
Black	280	410
Anglo	336	366

Source: Los Angeles County/University of Southern California Cancer Surveillance Program, presented at the American Cancer Society's Conference on Hispanics and Cancer, 1981.

Table 3. Incidence Rates per 100,000 for Cancers of Selected Sites Among Hispanic and Anglo Women

Geographic Area	Cancer Site	Hispanic	Anglo	Decrease Among Hispanics
Los Angeles	Breast	63	99	-36%
	Colon	19	32	-41%
	Lung	15	23	-35%
New Mexico	Breast	41	85	-52%
	Colon	15	29	-48%
	Lung	18	25	-28%
Texas	Breast	39	68	-43%
	Colon	15	29	-48%
	Lung	11	9	---

Anglo women for all three types of cancer. The decrease is similar in each area, ranging from about 30% to 50%. In determining different cancer rates among human groups, these would be considered large differences probably not accounted for by chance alone. As with other studies of cancer in human populations, these differences probably reflect environmental and/or life style influences more so than genetic or inherited factors.

Breast and colon cancers among Hispanic women were lower among those women who were not native born Americans and higher among those who were (Table 4). After migration, the occurrence of cancer usually assumes the higher rates common to the country of migration.[10] This again suggests environmental rather than genetic factors contributing to the cause(s) of these cancers.

For lung cancer, the overwhelming environmental cause is cigarette smoking. The challenge is to translate this knowledge into behavioral and societal attitudes that prevent young people from adopting cigarette smoking as a habit, and encourage habitual smokers to quit. For breast and colon cancers, the factors responsible for the differences are not known. The leading suspected life style factors for both sites is diet. Foods eaten may contain substances that cause the cancers to develop, on one hand, or that protect against their development on the other. Very few studies directed toward the relationship between diet and cancer among Hispanics have been conducted.

Table 4. Standardized Incidence Ratios (SIR)* for Mexican-Americans by Immigration Status, Los Angeles County, 1972-73 (5)

Cancer	Immigrant		Native	
Site	No.	SIR	No.	SIR
Breast	96	40	372	83
Colon	27	35	77	73
Lung	33	59	54	57

*SIR = Ratio of the incidence of the cancer by site to a standard incidence of 100. A ratio less than 100 indicates less cancer.

Economic Factors

Hispanics occupy a distinct position in the U.S. population and have experienced a different environment than other Americans. Hispanics are younger than the general U.S. population, and hold jobs of lower status.[5] Indicators of socioeconomic status show Hispanics to have lower incomes and less education compared to the total U.S. population (Table 5). No other ethnic group identified by the U.S. census has as high a fertility level as the Mexican-American, and the overall fertility rate combined with the typically large family size suggests a high risk for poorer maternal health.[3]

Nutritional Factors

Intermingling of Spanish and Indian cultures resulted in the adoption of the Indian culture of the New World based on the cultivation of corn. Because of this the subsequent diet of the Hispanic was based on corn and bean intake for protein. Using a 24-hour recall methodology, the Ten-State Nutrition Survey conducted between 1968 and 1970 concluded that almost one-third of low-income Hispanics reported no meat consumption and the highest legume and milk consumption of all groups studied.[11] In contrast, low-income Anglos reported the highest cereal and starch consumption.

In a study of adult Mexican Americans in Northern California, 53% worked in unskilled jobs and 81% had not graduated from high school (compared to 32% Anglos). Mexican-Americans used less low fat or skim milk (13 versus 28%) and more saturated fat for cooking (91 versus 67%). Mexican farm workers in California consumed a basically Mexican diet of beans and corn tortillas (pancakes) with some eggs, hamburgers, fruits, and rice with milk or gelatin desserts. They drank less coffee, beer, and tea, but more milk and soft drinks than Anglo families.[7]

Hispanic women attending prenatal clinics in Los Angeles county reported diets low in vitamin A, vitamin C and protein compared with all attendees. These diet histories were substantiated by measures of low blood vitamin C and low plasma levels of carotene, vitamin A and vitamin B_{12}.[7] Among Mexican Americans in Texas compared with all ethnic groups, low serum vitamin A and C and low plasma carotene levels were found.[11]

As noted previously, few studies of diet and cancer in Hispanic populations have been done, and those that were have been conducted in Hispanic groups other than those residing in this country. Thus, not only is dietary information about U.S. Hispanics sparse, but that which is available has not been linked to cancer occurrence among Hispanics. At this time, a plausible hypothesis for different occurrence of cancer in Hispanics may be differences in the diet. Whether these are related more to reduced intake of cancer-inducing sub-

Table 5. Selected Demographic and Socioeconomic Characteristics of Hispanics and Anglos (3)

Characteristic	Hispanic	Anglo
Median age, years	20.8	27.5
Percent native born	84.4	95.1
No. children/1000 15 to 24-year-old married women	1,264	933
Median year school completed	9.6	12.1
Mean family size	4.28	3.51
Mean family income ($)	8,550	11,348
Median family income ($)	7,533	9,957
% families under poverty level	20.4	8.6

stances or to an excess intake of protective substances, relative to Anglos, will be an exciting area of research for the future.

Breast Cancer

The incidence of breast cancer among women of three ethnic groups in Texas[8] is shown in Figure 1. The high rate of fertility and

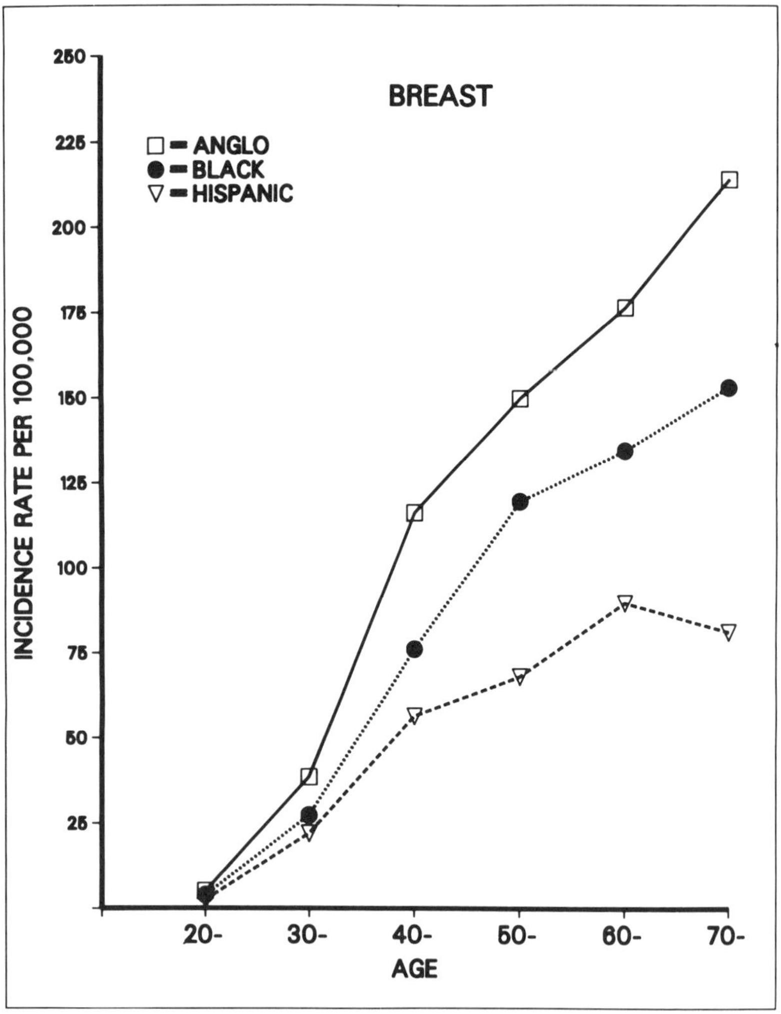

FIGURE 1. Breast Cancer in Hispanic, Black and Anglo Women, 1944–66. Source: Ref. 8.

reproductive habits of the Hispanic female, including marital status, pregnancy, and menstruation, may well protect her from the higher breast cancer risk experienced by her Anglo counterpart. In particular, there is a consistent pattern of protection conferred by early age of first pregnancy and multiple pregnancies. Women with first full-term pregnancies before age 20 had a relative risk of breast cancer one-third that of women whose first childbirth occurred after age 35. Of special interest was the fact that this relationship persisted after controlling for number of children, which is strongly related to age at first childbirth.

Demographic differences in ethnic groups are recognized, however, and within the Hispanic population in this country there is diversity in urban/rural residential patterns, socioeconomic levels, and other indicators of demographic status. The gradient in incidence rates from low in Texas to high in Los Angeles may reflect a more affluent, urbanized life style experienced by Hispanic females in Los Angeles.[3]

Various studies have implicated high intake of dietary fat with a higher incidence of breast cancer in Western countries. Various mechanisms have been proposed to explain the relationship between dietary fat and breast cancer, although to date none have been firmly established as etiologic factors in breast cancer. Increased intake of fat could influence endocrine metabolism and increase prolactin release from the pituitary gland or, by increasing bile salt production in the gut, lead to an altered bacterial flora and the production of carcinogenic substances.[12] However, one cannot say whether the lower breast cancer rates are due to lower amounts of fat consumption or higher intake of protective substances.

Colon Cancer

The incidence of colon cancer in males and females is shown in Figure 2. A lack of male/female difference suggests etiologic factors common to both sexes. There is some suggestion, although not strong, that cholecystectomy increases the risk of right-sided colon cancer. We recently interpreted this as not representing a cause and effect association.[13]

High ingestion of dietary fiber has been postulated to be protective against development of colon cancer. While several studies have investigated this theory, it is not yet clear whether it is the fiber itself or other protective factor(s) associated with fiber intake. Several studies have related the ingestion of vegetables, especially crucifers

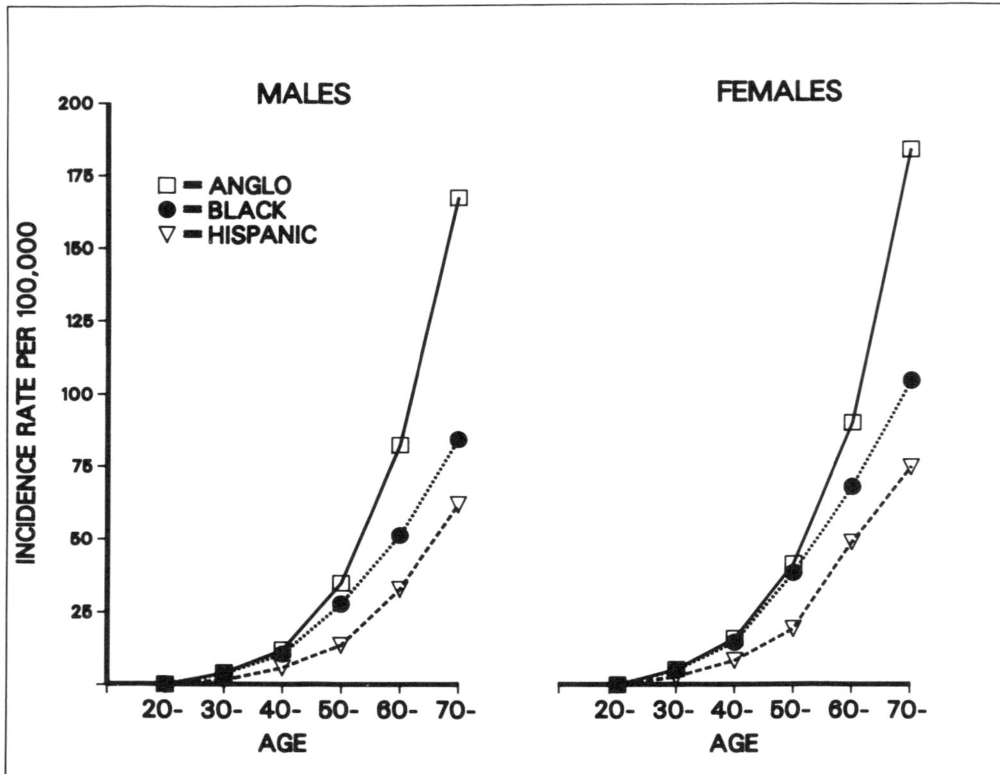

FIGURE 2. Colon Cancer in Hispanic, Black and Anglo Women and Men, 1944–66. Source: Ref. 8.

such as cabbage, broccoli and Brussels sprouts, with decreasing risk of colon cancer. These foods are known to be high in fiber. In addition, studies have compared Mormons in Utah and Seventh Day Adventists in California to the general populations in these same geographic areas. These studies showed major dietary differences between these groups and the general population and note lower cancer incidences for many sites, including breast and colon cancers.[14]

We currently have a large study underway to collect information on eating habits among the three ethnic groups in Texas. These actual measurements of food intake differences will be important in testing the proposed hypothesis.[4]

Lung Cancer

The pattern of occurrence of lung cancer is more complex than breast or colon cancers (Figure 3). There is a suggestion that lung cancer develops more often in older Hispanic women than younger ones. The same pattern has been reported for deaths from lung cancer among Hispanic women.[15] The suggestion was made that this may be due to heavier smoking among older Hispanic women who began smoking at a very early age during a time of social upheaval (during the Mexican Revolution of 1910). In addition, this cohort of migrant Mexican women may have been exposed to the custom of cooking over an open fire. A more plausible explanation is that this increase, if it is real, is probably due to error introduced because of misclassification. Nevertheless, the primary approach to reduce lung cancer in Hispanic women is the same as for Anglo women, namely the cessation of cigarette use. Recently, Hispanic women have been reported to smoke cigarettes less than their Anglo counterparts.[16]

CONCLUSIONS

In summary, Hispanic women in this country experience lower risk of developing and dying of cancers of the breast, colon and possibly lung than their Anglo counterparts. Although information on individual women is currently lacking—population-based statistics indicate that their lower breast cancer risk may be due, in part, to reproductive and menstrual experiences. Lower colon cancer rates may be attributable to the unique dietary habits of the Mexican-

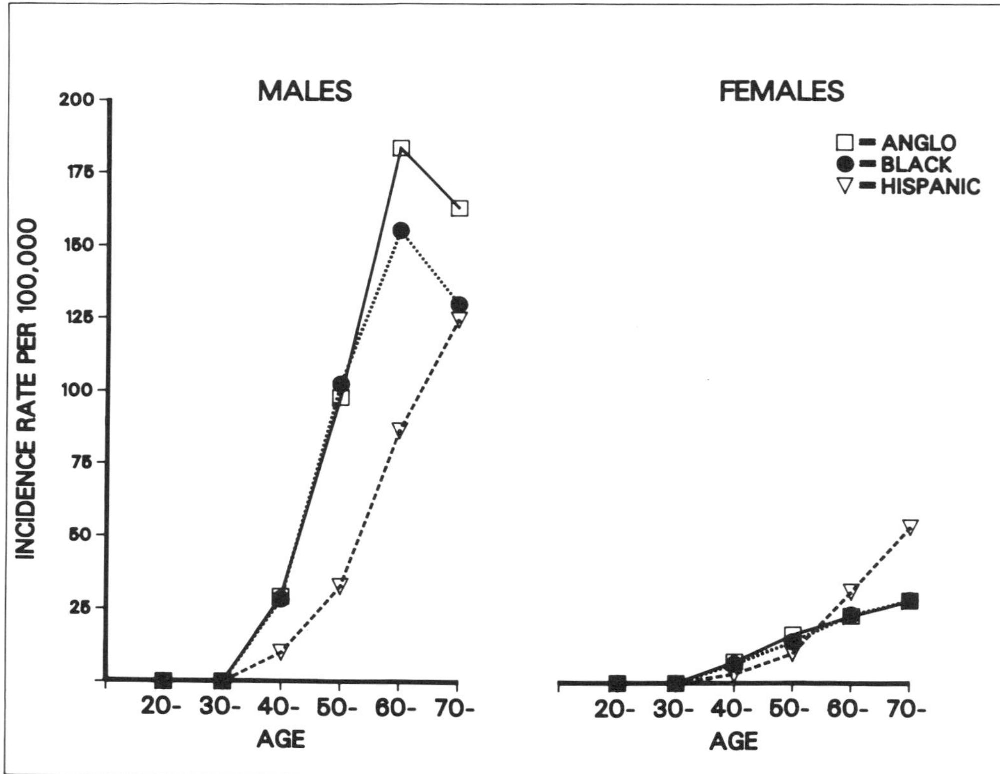

FIGURE 3. Lung Cancer in Hispanic, Black and Anglo Women and Men, 1944–66. Source: Ref. 8.

American women, particularly a traditional corn-based diet which may increase the level of dietary fiber in this group. The lower incidence of both breast and colon cancer may be due to the ingestion of protective substances in the Hispanic diet. There is a suggestion of less lung cancer among younger Hispanic than older ones. If so, it is probably due to differences in smoking patterns. The prevention of lung cancer in all groups rests with abstention or cessation of cigarette smoking.

NOTES

1. U.S. Department of Commerce (May 1978). Office of Federal Statistical Policy and Standards. Directory No. 15.

2. Young, J.L., Jr., Percy, C.L., & Asire, A.J. (eds). (1981). Surveillance, Epidemiology, and End Results: Incidence and Mortality Data, 1973–1977. *J Natl Cancer Inst Mono 57.*

3. Mills, P.K., & Newell, G.R. (1984). Epidemiology of breast cancer in Hispanics compared to Anglos. In *Current Controversies in Breast Cancer.* Ames, F.C., Blumenschein, G.R., & Montague E.D. (eds). University of Texas Press, Austin.

4. Newell, G.R., & Boutwell, W.B. (1981). Cancer differences among Texas ethnic groups—An hypothesis. *Cancer Bull* 33:113–114.

5. Menck, H.R., Henderson, B.E., Pike, M.C., et al. (1975). Cancer incidence in the Mexican-American. *J Natl Cancer Inst* 55:531–536.

6. U.S. Bureau of the Census, Statistical Abstract of the United States: 1984 (104th edition). (1983). Washington, D.C.

7. Lowenstein, F.W. (1981). Review of the nutritional status of Spanish Americans based on published and unpublished reports between 1968 and 1978. *Wld Rev Nutr Diet* 37:1–37.

8. Macdonald, E.J., & Heinze, E.B. (eds). (1978). Epidemiology of Cancer in Texas. Incidence Analyzed by Type, Ethnic Group, and Geographic Location. Raven Press, New York.

9. Hisserich, J.C., Martin, S.P., & Henderson, B.E. (1975). An area-wide cancer reporting network. *Public Hlth Rep* 90:15–18.

10. Kmet, J. (1970). The role of migrant population in studies of selected cancer sites: A review. *J Chr Dis* 23:305–324.

11. U.S. Dept. HEW. (1972). Ten-State Nutrition Survey, 1968–1970 (V Dietary). Publ No. (HSM) 72–813. Atlanta: Centers for Disease Control.

12. Wynder, E.L., McCoy, G.D., Reddy, B.S., Cohen, L., Hill, P., Spinagarn, N.E., & Weisburger, J.H. (1981). Nutrition and metabolic epidemiology of cancers of the oral cavity, esophagus, colon, breast, prostate, and stomach. In *Nutrition and Cancer: Etiology and Treatment*, pp. 11–48. Newell, G.R. and Ellison, N.M. (Eds). Raven Press, New York.

13. Spitz, M.R., Russell, N.C., Guinee, V.F., & Newell, G.R. (1985). Questionable relationship between cholecystectomy and colon cancer. *J Surg Onc.* 30:6–9.

14. Enstrom, J.E. (1980). Cancer mortality among Mormons in California during 1968–75. *J Natl Cancer Inst.* 65:1073–1082.

15. Lee, E.S., Roberts, R., & Labarthe, D.R. (1976). Excess and deficit lung cancer mortality in three ethnic groups in Texas. *Cancer* 38:2551–2556.

16. Holck, S.E., Warren, C., Rockat, R.W., & Smith, J.C. (1982). Lung cancer mortality and smoking habits: Mexican American women. *Amer J Public Health* 73:38–42.

Socioeconomic Status and Survival for Breast and Cervical Cancer

Donna P. Funch, PhD

ABSTRACT. This paper considers the association between socioeconomic status (SES) and survival from breast and cervical cancers, two major health problems for women. For both cancers, lower SES women appear to have poorer survival. Factors which may account for this are discussed, including biological and nutritional factors. Major emphasis is placed on early detection since this appears to play a critical role in the survival differential. Factors which act as barriers to early detection among poor women are considered, including those related both to the health behaviors of the poor and to the health care system available to the poor.

Among women in the U.S., two cancer sites, breast and cervix, account for almost one-third of all malignancies. Much of the research focus has been on identifying risk factors which could provide information for the primary prevention of these cancers. In the absence of clear etiologic factors, another interest has been in examining survival patterns for these sites to identify factors that play a role in secondary or tertiary prevention. During the past two decades a number of studies have found that racial and socioeconomic factors affect cancer survival rates. It is the goal of this paper to examine available data related to the role of socioeconomic status (SES) and cancer survival for these two sites and, more importantly, to try to identify specific factors which could account for poorer survival among the economically disadvantaged.

Donna P. Funch is with the Department of Social and Preventive Medicine, State University of New York at Buffalo, Buffalo, NY 14214.

This study was supported by the American Cancer Society grant no. JFRA-97 and by grant no. CA 11535 from the National Cancer Institute. Additional support was also received from the ACS subcommittee on Cancer Among the Economically Disadvantaged. The author would like to specially acknowledge the many helpful comments and suggestions from the following: Claudia Baquet, Susan Devesa, and C. David Jenkins.

SES AND CANCER SURVIVAL

This section will focus on the relation between SES and survival for breast and cervical cancer. The reader is referred to the article by Dr. Devesa in this issue for data on incidence and mortality trends for these sites. A number of the studies examing SES and survival do so using race as a proxy for SES since there is a strong association between race and SES in the United States, with blacks typically being located in lower socioeconomic categories. The relation between race, SES and survival will be discussed at a number of points in this paper.

It is interesting to note that cervical cancer has traditionally been associated with lower SES[1–3] while women with higher SES have been noted to be at increased risk for breast cancer.[4–6] Despite the opposing association between SES and incidence for these sites, survival is reduced for lower SES groups for both sites.

The five-year relative survival rates for the years 1960–81 for breast and cervical cancer are displayed in Figure 1 by race.[7] Relative survival rates have been used to adjust for differences in expected mortality due to other causes of death. Rates for 1960–73 are based on data from a series of hospital registries and one population-based registry. Rates for 1973–81 are from the Surveillance, Epidemiology and End Results (SEER) program which has a broader, more representative population. Data from these two sources are not strictly comparable but can be used to provide a general indication of changes in survival over time. Two points are clear from these data: (1) survival for both sites has improved over time for both races, particularly blacks; and (2) despite these improvements, the survival differential is apparent across time for both sites, although it is greatly reduced for cervical cancer.

While these data introduce the problem in a general way, they are limited to descriptive information on black-white trends. Tables 1 and 2 contain a summary of the studies which have specifically examined either SES[10–15] (Table 1) or black/white[16–20] (Table 2) survival differences. Research analyzing SES differences used primarily two measures of SES: (1) type of hospital providing care, generally public versus private[8,13] or (2) indirect measures of income or other SES-related factors based on median values of the census tract of residence.[10–12,14] A wide span of time is covered, ranging from 1940–1982. Most studies focused on five-year survival and utilized relative survival rates. The results of these studies

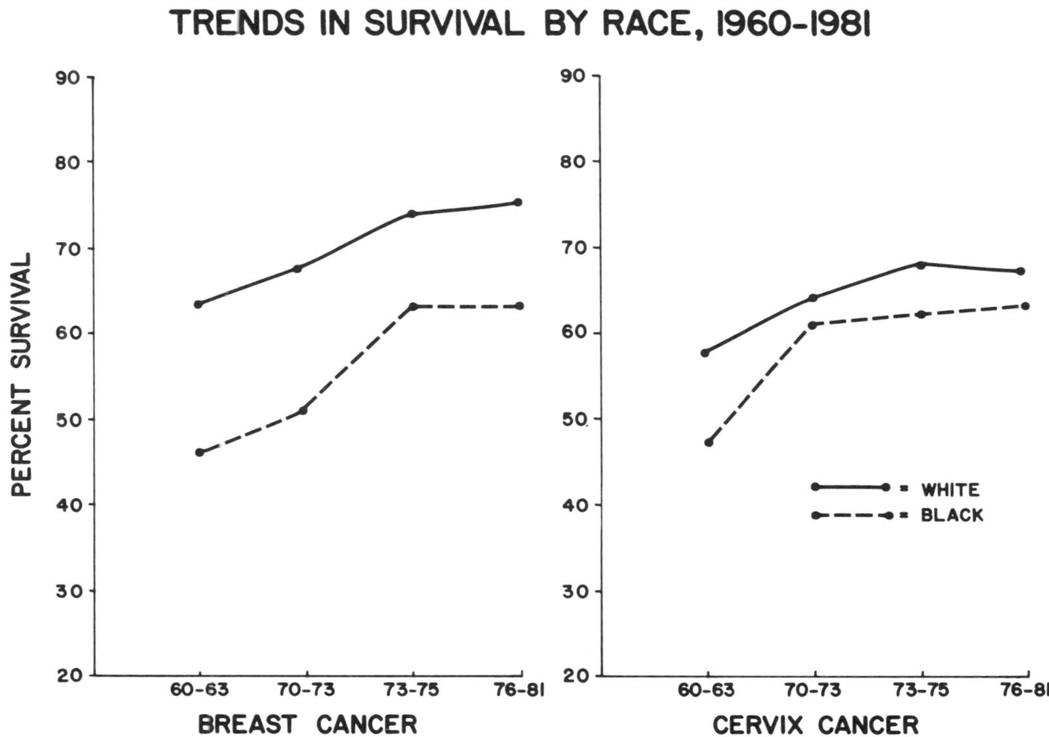

FIGURE 1. Trends in survival from breast cancer and cervix cancer for women, by calendar period and race, 1960–1981.

Table 1. Socioeconomic Status and Survival from Breast and Cervical Cancers

					Five-Year Relative Survival			
					All Stages		Localized Only	
Reference	SES Indicator	Time Period	Population	Site	High SES	Low SES	High SES	Low SES
8	Hospital type (private, clinic-pay, indigent)	1940-69	U. of Iowa Hospital Tumor Registry	Breast	54%	37%	--	--
				Cervix	73%	57%	--	--
13	Hospital type (public, private)	1942-56	California Tumor Registry (TR)	Breast	62%	35%	83%	67%
				Cervix	62%	39%	77%	78%
12	Census	1947-48	Chicago, Pittsburgh Dallas	Breast	47%	43%	66%	65%
				Cervix	43%	41%	62%	52%
11	Census	1959-63	New York (exclusive of NYC)	Cervix*	77%	71%	79%	75%
14	Census	1960-62	Connecticut	Breast**	71%	62%		
				Cervix**	70%	55%		
15	Years Educ.	1965-66	Boston	Breast	69%	52%		
10	Census, race	1968-77	Medical College of Virginia TR	Breast***	51%	37%		
9	census	1977-82	South Australia	Breast	78%	68%		
				Cervix	72%	60%		

*Percentages are calculated from a table.
**Three-year survival rates
***Percentages are estimated from a graph.

Table 2. Race and Survival from Breast and Cervical Cancers

Reference	Period	Population	Site	Five-Year Relative Survival: All Stages, Whites	All Stages, Blacks	Localized Only, Whites	Localized Only, Blacks
11	1955-64	End Results Group, NCI	Breast	62%	47%	84%	77%
			Cervix	60%	51%	79%	78%
17	1960-66	End Results Group, NCI	Breast	64%	47%	85%	78%
			Cervix	58%	46%	78%	74%
17	1967-73	Surveillance, Epidemiology, and End Results (SEER)	Breast	65%	51%	84%	81%
			Cervix	58%	53%	80%	77%
19	1963-73	Health Insurance Plan	Breast	61%	47%*		
20	1973-79	SEER, NCI	Breast	73%	61%	95%	91%
			Cervix	67%	62%		
18	1978	American College of Surgeons Survey	Breast	59%	47%	73%	71%

*Basec on a nonwhite, predominantly black sample

may be summarized as follows: (1) The majority of the studies looking at survival for all stages of disease show a positive association between SES and survival such that higher SES groups have greater survival. (2) Survival differences are present across all time periods. (3) In most cases, looking at localized cases only or adjusting statistically for stage differences results in a reduction of the survival differential, suggesting that differences in stage at diagnosis by SES play a role in survival. (4) The pattern for blacks is similar to that for lower SES groups in general, suggesting that, at least for these two sites, racial differences are basically a function of SES. This is also directly supported by two studies, one looking at breast cancer only and the other at breast and cervical cancer.[10,13] Both studies had information on SES and race; SES appeared to be the predominant factor influencing survival.

FACTORS RELATED TO SURVIVAL

These data suggest that for these two sites survival differences do exist based on SES. Assuming SES does affect survival, the next step is to determine possible causal mechanisms. One of the major explanations offered for these survival differences is related to stage of disease at diagnosis, a variable known to be highly associated with survival. Enterline and Gold[21] point out that stage represents one component of survival which is amenable to secondary prevention through early detection. Early detection is a realistic possibility for the two sites of interest here since effective techniques have been identified to detect breast and cervical cancers early in their development.[14,22,23] This is particularly true for cervical cancer where the frequency of *in situ* cancer is directly dependent upon the availability and utilization of cervical smears and detection at the precancerous stage can halt the progression of the disease with a minor operation.[3,24] If late detection accounts for at least some of the survival difference for these two sites, one would expect to see a relation between SES and stage. In fact, one does find more advanced disease among lower SES groups for both breast[25,26] and cervical cancer.[8,11,12,14] Blacks also tend to be diagnosed with more advanced disease.[17,25,27–30]

One may roughly estimate the extent to which early detection could reduce the survival difference by comparing survival differences for all stages versus those for localized disease only. This can be done with the information presented in the right-hand columns of Tables 1 and 2. For example, in the second study listed in Table 1,[13] there is 27% difference in five-year survival for breast cancer between high and low SES women which is reduced to 16% if only localized cancers are considered. For cervical cancer the initial difference of 23% is completely eliminated with early detection. With the exception of the Haenszel and Chiazze study[12] in which no significant differences in survival by SES were observed, both sites consistently show some reduction in the survival differential when stage is taken into account.

Breast and cervical cancers display slightly different patterns when looking at stage effects. For breast cancer, stage of disease at diagnosis failed to account for all of the observed difference in survival. A number of studies found elevated survival for higher SES groups and for whites which persisted even after adjusting for stage.[8,10,13,18,20,29,30] Some have suggested that this residual SES effect may partially be a result of variation existing within each staging category which is not accounted for by the use of broad categories such as local, regional and distant. Recent SEER data (1975–81) containing more detailed staging information found survival differences between blacks and whites were minimal (3–4%) when considering the smallest tumors with no nodal involvement.[31] There is also some additional evidence for the important role of early detection. In one investigation, members of a prepaid group practice were randomly assigned to either a control group, receiving standard medical care, or a screening group who were offered an initial breast screening exam together with three additional annual follow-up exams.[19] Of the women in the control group who developed breast cancer, 5-year survival rates were significantly different for nonwhites (47%) versus whites (61%). Survival rates were almost identical between races for the screening group (nonwhites-77%; whites-73%). This study together with the SEER data suggest that when breast cancers are detected at the earliest stage, the difference between races is minimal or nonexistent.

The survival difference for cervical cancer is generally smaller between SES groups than that for breast cancer, especially when localized cancers are considered. Black/white differences in survival are also much smaller when stage is taken into account.[16,17,32] Two studies specifically examined the relation between SES and survival from cervical cancer and found a significant positive association which was either greatly reduced[8] or eliminated[11] among cancers with no spread. The time trends for survival for blacks and whites presented in Figure 1 also may provide indirect support for the role of early detection as an important component in the survival differential. For the years 1960–63 there is an 11% difference in survival between blacks and whites which is rapidly reduced to 3% by the years 1970–73 and maintained at a low level thereafter. This coincides with the general introduction of cytologic screening programs in the 1960s which played a major role in the detection of cervical cancer at a very early, treatable stage.

Taken together, these findings support the potentially major role which early detection may play for both cervical and breast cancer. Other factors may also be operating to reduce survival among disadvantaged groups. Because of the black/white differences in survival, which in some cases are maintained even with adjustment for SES, some have suggested there may be underlying biological differences between the two races. This seems unlikely however since risk factors are the same for both races,[4] suggesting the underlying disease process is similar. Racial differences in survival may remain despite adjustment for SES because the relatively crude categories of SES may fail to adequately discriminate various SES levels for blacks. In addition, even when SES indicators are technically equivalent, such as when both blacks and whites have a high school education, the type and quality of the education received may vary for these groups. Even if SES could be accurately accounted for, however, some recent data on other ethnic groups raise additional questions. Hispanic women have survival rates similar to whites for both breast and cervical cancer although their SES level is similar to that of blacks.[20] This does not appear to be due to differences in treatment-seeking; at least one study has noted that both black and Hispanic women tend to delay seeking care.[29] Comparative studies of this type may provide valuable information on cultural factors that may influence survival.

Nutrition may also play a role in cancer survival. Considerable emphasis has been placed on the tendency for lower SES groups to be diagnosed with later stage tumors. The assumption often made is that, for one reason or another, these people delay in seeking care or are unable to get attention for their problem early enough. While these are real possibilities, it is also possible that factors such as nutrition could play a role in reducing one's resistance to a cancer or otherwise promote growth so that a tumor initiated in a lower SES woman at the same time as one in a higher SES women would more rapidly reach an advanced stage. Karp and Greene have pointed out that there is little margin for error or waste in the diets of the poor and increasing food costs frequently cause marginal diets to become deficient in micronutrients.[33] Some of these micronutrients are thought to play a protective role in cancer initiation or promotion.[34]

Poor nutrition may also have a direct impact on treatment success and survival. Some studies have found a correlation between nutritional status at initial examination and response to treatment.[35] Inadequate nutrition can impair host immune responses and can also increase the risk of infections.[35] Individuals who are compromised in terms of nutritional status in general could have even more difficulty during the treatment process when the cancer itself, and sometimes the treatment as well, may lead to additional malnutrition.[36] Prospective studies of the relation between nutritional status and prognosis in terms of treatment response, incidence of complications, relapse rates and survival are needed.[35] More information will be necessary to determine thresholds of malnutrition which are of clinical significance with respect to cancer promotion and survival.[37] Should nutrition prove to be an important factor, one will need to consider how best to alter the nutrional status of the poor. Lower SES groups appear to have less knowledge of nutritional factors, which could affect their food choices.[38] Even if their knowledge of nutrition is increased, however, food costs might inhibit the purchase of nutritious foods.[33,39,40]

Factors which operate following treatment may also play a role in survival. Aspects of the social or economic environment of the poor may limit the ability of the family to care of the patient.[41] Poor patients may also fail to obtain appropriate health care services following surgery, including regular follow-up examinations.[42] More data are needed in these areas.

EARLY DETECTION PROBLEMS FOR THE DISADVANTAGED

A number of possible factors affecting cancer survival among the disadvantaged have been noted. Probably one of the most important and identifiable of these factors is early detection. Because of the important role which this factor plays, this section will briefly discuss some of the limitations connected with achieving a rapid increase in early detection among the poor.

The best opportunity to detect cancer is through screening exams where cancer can be detected at the asymptomatic or pre-clinical point. For both breast and cervical cancer screening tests have been developed for this purpose.[22] In order for these tests to increase the percentage of cancers detected early in poor women, the tests must be available to that segment of the population. It is apparent, however, that simply increasing the availability of screening facilities alone will not improve survival among the poor. Women most in need of these services are least likely to use them.[43,44] A number of major screening programs, including some aimed specifically at lower SES black populations, have attracted disproportionate numbers of higher SES women.[45–47] One breast cancer screening study used central Harlem as the target population because of the extremely large percentage of women diagnosed with advanced breast cancer in that area. Despite massive media coverage, they got only a fraction of the number of screenees they hoped for and only 20% of those came from the target area.[45]

The failure of poor women to take full advantage of screening programs may partially result from lower levels of knowledge regarding cancer,[48] and also from a general lack of orientation towards prevention.[49] Cancer education programs have been developed to address this problem. While women in general are more likely to use these services, poor women use them less frequently than other women.[50,51]

One method for increasing the use of preventive health services may be through involvement of members of the local community in the educational process.[52] "Word of mouth" information from family and friends was found to improve participation in screening programs.[45] In one study residents of a black community were trained to provide information to other members of the community on both the value of early detection and the availability of programs providing these services.[53] Contact with these health aides was the most important factor leading to use of these services; information transmitted via impersonal media was the least effective. Other studies also support the value of "indigenous" health workers, noting that communication between these workers and poor clients is much more effective than between the poor and middle or upper class professionals.[23,54] There may, however, be some problems associated with the use of these workers due to such factors as: (1) insufficient training; (2) the failure to be accepted as "expert" enough by the patients; and (3) reduced effectiveness over time as the workers increasingly come to identify with the professionals.[54] More research examining various mechanisms for community involvement in health promotion is necessary to identify those methods which most effectively address the needs of the community.

Even when lower SES clients are attracted to screening clinics, they are more likely to drop out of these programs. The Breast Cancer Detection Demonstration Project had only a small number of black women and they tended to drop out after only one or two screenings. Lower levels of income and education were also associated with dropping out,[46] even among women with positive findings.[43,55] It is clear, therefore, that simply removing economic deterrents is not sufficient,[49] and it is likely that effective educational strategies need to be linked with direct and relatively uncomplicated access to screening and other early detection programs. It is also important to recognize the need to educate health care workers to the special needs and orientations of different socioeconomic and cultural subgroups so that they can respond more effectively in providing health care services.

It may be important for the poor to receive prevention-oriented screening, like pap smears and breast exams, as an automatic part of a physical exam or during visits for the treatment of other non-related problems.[25] The average number of visits to a physician per year is similar for various racial and economic subgroups.[56] Data on the use of selected medical procedures associated with preventive care (e.g., pap smears, breast exams), however, suggest that non-whites and lower SES groups are less likely to receive these procedures. For example, in one national survey, 35% of the women in the lowest income group had never received a breast exam versus 13% of women in the highest income group. For pap smears the comparable figures were 39% versus 15%.[56] This is consistent with other work suggesting that the preventive health practices of physicians vary with the SES of the populations they serve.[26] Because black patients and other lower SES groups may rely more heavily on clinics than on private physicians, clinics will need to be more systematically organized for the provision of screening exams and will also need mechanisms for patient follow-up and education.[49]

It is generally agreed that diagnosing breast and cervical cancer in the asymptomatic woman through screening offers the best possibility for early detection. There is also some evidence,[57–60] although not totally consistent,[61,62] suggesting that prompt treatment-seeking in the symptomatic woman with breast cancer may still result in detection of cancer at earlier stages and improve survival. A number of studies have noted that women with lower levels of education and income are less likely to practice breast self-examination and are more likely to delay.[63–68] Both of these practices may be partially a function of the type of health care available to the poor. Having a regular source of care appears to play a role in both patient education and timely treatment-seeking.[43,69] A significantly larger portion of the economically disadvantaged use hospital emergency rooms as their primary source of medical care.[70] Persons who use emergency rooms as opposed to primary care sources have been found to delay more when experiencing a cancer symptom.[68] Emergency rooms are geared for the treatment of apparently sick people and a minimally symptomatic patient is likely to be discouraged.[71]

Taken together, these comments suggest that early detection may be an important mechanism for reducing the survival differential between lower and higher SES groups for cervical and breast cancers. It is also clear, however, that there are many factors operating which stand in the way of increasing early detection for lower SES women, and men as well. We need to have a better understanding of the barriers, both real and perceived, to the poor in obtaining prompt, effective health care. We also need to learn more about the attitudes and practices of those health professionals who serve the poor and about the constraints placed on them by the current medical care system.

SUGGESTIONS FOR FUTURE RESEARCH

This paper has compared breast and cervical cancer survival among different economic groups and identified differences in survival. Several factors were mentioned which might play a role in the reduced survival among the poor. A number of questions have been raised which deserve more study. This final section will focus on a few of the key questions that remain.

First, there are a number of issues related to the measurement of SES and the limitations on our knowledge implied by the crude measures generally employed. As noted in this paper, SES has frequently been used categorically, often dividing samples into low and high SES groups. This practice has resulted, in part, from the limitations of the SES measures themselves. Generally subjects have been classified based either on the type of hospital they received their treatment from or on socioeconomic data relevant to the general area they live in, rather than on any personal information on SES. The limitations in working with these types of indirect measures have generally confined investigators to classifying subjects in broad SES groupings. This has restricted the hypotheses which can be considered. For example, while lower SES groups generally appeared to have poorer survival for both sites, one could not consider at what point on the SES scale these reductions in expected survival actually begin or what shape the survival curve takes as a function of SES. Some studies with information on lower, middle, and upper SES groups have noted, for example, that middle and upper SES groups have similar survival.[29,72] There may be a threshold effect such that only patients with economic status below a given level suffer reductions in survival. The use of gross SES categories makes it impossible to consider a threshold hypothesis and, along with this, makes it more difficult to identify high risk populations which may be of particular interest to cancer control programs.

While measurement problems limit our ability to analyze more accurately the relation between SES and cancer survival, they may not be critical to our understanding of the factors involved in the survival differential. SES factors like education and income are only acting as surrogates in the survival analyses. It is likely that they are representing more specific risk-related behaviors such as limited access to screening, patient delay, and poor nutrition. For some of these, such as nutrition, very little information is available on SES differences; for others, such as patient delay, we know the behavior is related to SES but not enough research has been done to determine *how* SES is associated with delay.

Considerable attention has been given to issues surrounding early detection since this appears to play a major role in reducing the survival differential between groups and generally increases survival for all women with these cancers. It has been noted that screening programs appear to have difficulty reaching the members of the population who are at greatest risk. Some research has already suggested that there are differences between groups regarding the types of media most effective in promoting programs and educating the public directly.[50,73–76] More research is needed to identify effective educational strategies, possibly involving multimedia approaches and targeting programs for specific populations. A number of studies have identified the role which family and friends play in providing information and support for the use of early detection services. How can these informal networks best be mobilized? Lower SES groups, especially blacks, seem to be less likely to receive screening procedures as part of their routine visits to their health care providers. Why does this situation exist and what can be done to change it? Can programs be developed which effectively combine visits to the medical care system for specific problems with health promotion and early detection procedures? Once an individual is brought into the medical care system for screening, what techniques are most effective in keeping that person actively involved? Once a problem has been identified (e.g. detection of a lump or abnormal cervical smear), what measures can be used to assure adequate follow-up of that problem?

In this report, very little attention has been given to factors, other than those related to early detection, which may affect survival following diagnosis. Do poor women receive different treatment than women with greater economic resources? Are certain types of treatment less effective for the disadvantaged? What role does the general nutritional status of the patient play in treatment effectiveness and what levels of malnutrition reach clinical significance? What role does the home environment of the poor play in recovery? A number of studies have suggested that social support is important but we know very little about the support networks of the poor. What factors are associated with noncompliance with respect to treatments (e.g. chemotherapy) and routine follow-up examinations? To what extent is rehabilitative treatment available to the poor? What is the quality of survival for the poor?

SUMMARY

Women who are economically disadvantaged appear to have poorer survival from breast and cervical cancer despite general improvements over time. One major factor which appears to play a role in the disparity in survival is the failure of poor women to be diagnosed as often in the early stages of disease. This problem appears to be a complex one which cannot be solved simply by increasing the availability of screening services. It was noted that poor women are less likely to know about screening techniques, less likely to use them, less likely to get appropriate follow-up examinations for positive test results, and more likely to delay treatment-seeking once they become symptomatic. All of these behaviors contribute to later detection of disease and the resulting reduction in survival associated with it. Other factors more common among the disadvantaged, such as malnutrition, competing illnesses, and an impoverished home environment, may also influence survival. Additional research is needed to determine both the role of these factors and how they may best be modified to improve survival. Because many different factors may be involved in determining cancer outcomes, this problem offers an opportunity to researchers from a variety of disciplines to work together to identify acceptable and effective methods for improving survival for everyone.

NOTES

1. Cuello, C., Correa, P. & Haenszel, W. (1982). Socio-economic class differences in cancer incidence in Cali, Columbia. *Int. J. Cancer*, 29:637–643.

2. Devesa, S.S., & Diamond, E.L. (1980). Association of breast cancer and cervical cancer incidence with income and education among whites and blacks. *J. Natl. Cancer Inst.*, 65:515–528.

3. Morton, W.E., Baker, H.W., & Fletcher, W.S. (1983). Geographic pathology of uterine cancers in Oregon: Risks of double primaries and effects of socioeconomic status. *Gyn. Oncol.*, 16:63–77.

4. Austin, H., Cole, P., & Wynder, E. (1979). Breast cancer in black American women. *Int. J. Cancer*, 24:541–544.

5. Talamini, R., LaVecchia, C., Decarli, A., Franceschi, S., Grattoni, E., Grigoletto, E., Liberati, A., & Tognoni, G. (1984). Social factors, diet and breast cancer in a Northern Italian population. *Br. J. Ca.*, 49:723–729.

6. Williams, R.R., & Horm, J.W. (1977). Association of cancer sites with tobacco and alcohol consumption and socioeconomic status of patients: Interview study from the Third National Cancer Survey. *J. Natl. Ca. Inst.*, 58:525–547.

7. American Cancer Society. (1985). Cancer Statistics, 1985. *CA—A Cancer Journal for Clinicians*, 35:19–35.

8. Berg, J.W., Ross, R., & Latourette, H.B. (1977). Economic status and survival of cancer patients. *Cancer*, 39:467–477.

9. Bonett, A., Roder, D., & Esterman, A. (1984). Determinants of case survival for cancers of the lung, colon, breast and cervix in South Australia. *Med. J. Aust.*, 141:705–709.

10. Dayal, H.H., Povver, R.N., & Chiu, C. (1982). Race and socioeconomic status in survival from breast cancer. *J. Chron. Dis.*, 35:675–683.

11. Graham, S., Priore, R.L., Schueller, E.F., & Burnett, W. (1972). Epidemiology of survival from cancer of the cervix. *J. Natl. Ca. Inst.*, 49:639–647.

12. Haenszcl, W., & Chiazze, L.J. (1965). Survival experience of cancer patients enumerated in morbidity surveys. *J. Natl. Ca. Inst.*, 34:85–101.

13. Linden, G. (1969). The influence of social class in the survival of cancer patients. *Am. J. Publ. Hlth.*, 59:267–274.

14. Lipworth, L., Abelin, T., & Connelly, R.R. (1970). Socioeconomic factors in the prognosis of cancer patients. *J. Chron. Dis.*, 23:105–116.

15. Morrison, A.S., Lowe, C.R., MacMahon, B., Ravnihar, B., & Yuasa S. (1977).

Incidence risk factors and survival in breast cancer: Report on five years of follow-up observation. *Europ. J. Cancer*, 13:209–214.

16. Axtell, L.M., Myers, M.H., & Shambaugh, E.M. (1975). Treatment and survival patterns for black and white cancer patients diagnosed 1955 through 1964. DHEW Pub. No. (NIH) 75–712, 1–41.

17. Axtell, L.M., & Myers, M.H. (1978). Contrasts in survival of black and white cancer patients, 1960–75. *J. Natl. Ca. Inst.*, 60:1209–1215.

18. Nemoto, T., Vana, J., Bedwani, R.N., Baker, H., McGregor, F.H., & Murphy, G.P. (1980). Management and survival of female breast cancer: Results of a national survey by the American College of Surgeons. *Cancer*, 45:2917–2924.

19. Shapiro, S., Venet, W., Strax, P., Venet, L., & Roeser, R. (1982). Prospects for eliminating racial differences in breast cancer survival rates. *Am. J. Pub. Hlth.*, 72:1142–1145.

20. Young, J.L., Jr., Ries, L.G., & Pollack, E.S. (1984). Cancer patient survival among ethnic groups in the United States. *J. Natl. Ca. Inst.*, 73:341–352.

21. Enterline, J.P., & Gold, E.B. (1983). A method for estimating the potential effects of primary and secondary prevention activities in high risk populations. In *Progress in Cancer Control IV: Research in the Cancer Center*. New York: Alan R. Liss.

22. Cairns, J. (1985). The treatment of diseases and the war against cancer. *Scientific American*, 253:51–59.

23. Green, L.W. (1978). Determining the impact and effectiveness of health education as it relates to federal policy. *Hlth. Ed. Monog.*, (Suppl 1) 6:28–66.

24. Fielding, J.E. (1978). Successes of Prevention. *Mil. Mem. Fund. Q.*, 56:274–302.

25. Howard, J. (1982). In-Reach: An approach to the secondary prevention of cancer. In Behavior, Health Risks, and Social Disadvantage (Parron, D.L., Solomon, F., & Jenkins, C.D., Eds.). Washington, DC: National Academy Press.

26. Howard, J., Lund, P., & Bell, G. (1980). Hospital variations in metastatic breast cancer. *Med. Carc*, 18:442–455.

27. Lewison, E.F., Montague, A.C., & Kuller, L. (1966). Breast cancer treated at the Johns Hopkins Hospital, 1951–56. *Cancer*, 19:1359–1368.

28. Potter, J.F., Terry, P., Dawkins, D.M., & Bievers, D.G. (1983). Breast cancer in blacks, Asians, and whites in Birmingham. *Postgrad. Med. J.*, 59:661–663.

29. Vernon, S.W., Tilley, B.C., Neale, A.V., & Steinfeldt, L. (1985). Ethnicity, survival, and delay in seeking treatment for symptoms of breast cancer. *Cancer*, 55:1563–1571.

30. Walker, A.R.P., Walker, B.F., Tshabalala, E.N., Isaacson, C., & Segal, I. (1984). Low survival of South African urban black women with breast cancer. *Br. J. Ca.*, 49:241–244.

31. National Cancer Advisory Board. (1984). Annual Cancer Statistics Review. Prepared by Demographic Analysis Section, Biometry Branch, Division of Cancer Prevention and Control, NCI.

32. American Cancer Society. (1984). Cancer Facts and Figures—1984. *CA—A Cancer Journal for Clinicians*, 31:7–23.

33. Karp, R., & Greene, G.W. (1983). The effect of rising food costs on the occurrence of malnutrition among the poor in the United States: The Engels Phenomenon in 1983. *Bull. N.Y. Acad. Med.*, 59:721–727.

34. Yuspa, S.H. (1983). Retinoids and tumor promotion. *Current Topics in Nutrition and Disease*, 9:95–109.

35. Nutritional Reviews. (1982). Nutritional status of cancer patients. *Nutritional Reviews*, 40:263–265.

36. Dickerson, J.W.T. (1984). Nutrition in the cancer patient: A review. *J. Royal Soc. Med.*, 77:309–315.

37. Chandra, R.K. (1983). Nutrition, immunity, and infection: Present knowledge and future directions. *Lancet*, (8326) 1:688–691.

38. Rahn, M.J., & Sabry, J.H. (1984). Nutrition knowledge of a sample of urban women. *Am. J. Pub. Hlth.*, 75:123–127.

39. Fox, B.H. (1984) Remote life-style causes of cancer. *Cancer Det. Prev.*, 7:21–29.

40. Gori, G.B. (1979). Dieting and nutritional implications in the multifactorial etiology of certain prevalent human cancers. *Cancer*, 43:2151–2161.

41. Feldman, J.G., Gardner, B., Carter, A.C., Alfonso, A., & Orces, H. (1979). Relation of race to functional status among breast cancer patients after curative surgery. *J. Surg. Oncol.*, 11:333–339.

42. Funch, D., & Mettlin, C. (1982). The role of support in relation to recovery from breast surgery. *Soc. Sci. Med.*, 16:91–98.

43. Greenwald, H.P., Becker, S.W., & Newitt, M.C. (1978). Delay and noncompliance in cancer detection. *Mil. Mem. Fund Q.*, 56:212–230.

44. Helsing, K.J., & Comstock, G.W. (1978). Psychosocial characteristics and cytologic screening for cervical cancer. *Prev. Med.*, 7:550–560.

45. Adams, M., Kerner, J.F. (1982). Evaluation of promotional strategies to solve the problem of underutilization of a breast examination/education center in a New York City black community. In *Issues in Cancer Screening and Communications* (Mettlin, C., & Murphy, G.P., Eds.). New York: Alan R. Liss, pp. 151–161.

46. Baker, L.H. (1982). Breast Cancer Detection Demonstration Project: Five year summary report. *CA—A Cancer Journal for Clinicians*, 32:194–225.

47. Grover, P.L., Prakash, L., Kulpa, B., Sampson, B.T., & Engstrom, P.F. (1982). Role of education in screening for cancer control: Results of follow up in two screening programs. In *Issues in Cancer Screening and Communications* (Mettlin, C., Murphy, G.P.). New York: Alan R. Liss, pp. 231–247.

48. Hill, L.T. (1982). Cancer—the behavioral dimension. An interaction of lifestyle and disease. In *Behavior, Health Risks, and Social Disadvantage* (Parron, D.L., Solomon, F., & Jenkins, C.D., Eds.). Washington D.C.: National Academy Press.

49. Warnecke, R.B. (1981). Intervention in black populations. In *Cancer Among Black Populations*. New York: Alan R. Liss, pp. 167–183.

50. Parker, D.F., Enterline, J.P., & White, J.E. (1982). Differences between black and white responses to cancer information service promotion mechanisms. In *Issues in Cancer Screening and Communications* (Mettlin, C., & Murphy, G.P., Eds.). New York: Alan R. Liss, pp. 429–436.

51. Wilkinson, G.S., & Wilson, J. (1983). An evaluation of demographic differences in the utilization of a cancer information service. *Soc. Sci. Med.*, 17:169–175.

52. Kupchik, G.J. (1969). Environmental health in the ghetto. *Am. J. Publ. Hlth.*, 59:220–225.

53. Warnecke, R.B., Graham, S., Mosher, W., Montgomery, E., Schotz, W.E., et al. (1975). Contact with health guides and use of health services among an inner-city population. *Publ. Hlth. Rep.*, 90:213–222.

54. Grosser, C.F. (1966). Local residents as mediators between middle-class professional workers and lower-class clients. *Soc. Serv. Rev.*, 40:56–63.

55. Michielutte, R., Diseker, R.A., Young, L.D., & May, W.J. (1985). Noncompliance in screening follow-up among family planning clinic patients with cervical dysplasia. *Prev. Med.*, 14:248–258.

56. United States Department of Health, Education and Welfare. (1977). Use of selected medical procedures associated with preventive care, United States—1973. DHEW Pub. No. (HRA) 77–1538.

57. Anglem, T.J., & Leber, R.E. (1971). Characteristics of ten year survivors after radical mastectomy for cancer of the breast. *Am. J. Surg.*, 121:363–367.

58. Brinkley, D., & Haybittle, J.L. (1968). A 15-year follow-up study of patients treated for carcinoma of the breast. *Br. J. Radiol.*, 41:215–221.

59. Elwood, J.M., & Moorehead, W.P. (1980). Delay in diagnosis and long-term survival in breast cancer. *Br. Med. J.*, 280:1291–1294.

60. Huguley, C.M., & Brown, R.L. (1981). The value of breast self-examination. *Cancer* 47:989–995.

61. Dennis, C.R., Gardner, B., & Lim, B. (1975). Analysis of survival and recurrence versus patient and doctor delay in treatment of breast cancer. *Cancer*, 35:714–720.

62. Fisher, E.R., Redmond, C., & Fisher, B. (1977). A perspective concerning the relation of duration of symptoms to treatment failure in patients with breast cancer. *Cancer*, 40:3160–3167.

63. Blackwell, B. (1983). The literature of delay in seeking medical care for chronic illness. *Hlth. Ed. Monog.*, 16:3–31.

64. Cameron, A., & Hinton, J. (1968). Delay in seeking treatment for mammary tumors. *Cancer*, 21:1121–1126.

65. Funch, D.P. (1984). The role of patient delay in the evaluation of breast self-examination. *J. Psychosoc. Oncol.*, 2:31–39.

66. Greer, S. (1974). Psychological aspects: Delay in the treatment of breast cancer. *Proc. Roy. Soc. Med.*, 67:470–473.

67. Howe, H.L. (1981). Social factors associated with breast self-examination among high risk women. *Am. J. Pub. Hlth.*, 71:251–255.

68. Gould-Martin, K., Paganini-Hill, A., Casagrande, C., Mack, R., & Ross, R.K. (1982). Behavioral and biological determinants of surgical stage of breast cancer. *Prev. Med.*, 11:429–440.

69. Steinwachs, D.M., & Yaffe, R. (1978). Assessing the timeliness of ambulatory medical care. *Am. J. Pub. Hlth.*, 68:547–556.

70. Haughton, J.G., & DasGuptas, T.K. (1979). Meeting the crisis of health care delivery to black Americans in urban centers. Proceedings of the ACS National Conference on Meeting the Challenge of Cancer Among Black Americans. New York: American Cancer Society.

71. Lefall, L. (1981). Program priorities for the future. *Prog. Clin. Biol. Res.*, 53:253–263.

72. LeMarchand, L., Kolonel, L.N., & Nomura, A.M.Y. (1984). Relation of ethnicity and other prognostic factors to breast cancer survival patterns in Hawaii. *J. Natl. Ca. Inst.*, 73:1259–1265.

73. Butler, L., King, G., & White, J. (1983). Communications strategies, cancer information and black populations: An analysis of longitudinal data. Progress in Cancer Control IV: Research in the Cancer Center. New York: Alan R. Liss, pp. 171–182.

74. Denniston, R.W. (1981). Cancer knowledge, attitudes, and practices among black Americans. In *Cancer Among Black Populations*. New York: Alan R. Liss, pp. 225–235.

75. Michielutte, R., Diseker, R.A. (1982). Racial differences in knowledge of cancer. *Soc. Sci. Med.*, 16:245–252.

76. Putman, G.L, Brannon, B., & Yanagisako, K.L. (1982). Multimedia public/professional skin cancer education in a multiethnic setting. In *Issues in Cancer Screening and Communications* (Mettlin, C., & Murphy, G.P., Eds.). New York: Alan R. Liss, pp. 437–448.

Breast Self-Examination Among College Females

B. Jo Hailey, PhD

ABSTRACT. Self-reported behavior and attitudes toward breast self-examination (BSE) among 230 female college students age 20 and older revealed that less than one in four were compliant with American Cancer Society recommendations of monthly practice. Respondents were classified as examiners (N = 113) if they reported BSE practice at least 6 times a year. A discriminant analysis produced a significant degree of separation between examiners and non-examiners ($\chi^2(3) = 90.199, p < .005$) and identified three variables which significantly discriminated the groups. Examiners were (a) more familiar with BSE, (b) more worried about cancer, and (c) more willing to increase their knowledge about BSE. Initial exposure to BSE was from physicians or print media; however, subjects expressed a preference for learning more about the technique in a person-to-person setting with another woman or women. Respondents reported that reminders would be likely to increase BSE frequency.

Breast cancer will afflict about 123,000 women in 1986 and take the lives of nearly 40,000 (American Cancer Society, 1986). It is the leading cause of cancer death among women 15–54, and will strike one out of every eleven women at sometime during her life (Silverberg and Lubera, 1986). Since little is known about effective ways to prevent breast cancer, early detection and treatment are extremely important determinants of survival.

Breast self-examination (BSE) and mammography are two major components of an effective early detection program. The American Cancer Society recommends the monthly practice of BSE by women 20 years and older (American Cancer Society, 1986). Several reports indicate that regular practice of BSE leads to earlier discovery of cancer and longer survival. Foster et al. (1978) studied 355 patients with breast cancer, and found that more frequent performance of BSE

Requests for reprints should be addressed to B. Jo Hailey, Department of Psychology, University of Southern Mississippi, Southern Station, Box 9371, Hattiesburg, MS 39406.

was associated with more favorable clinical stage and fewer axillary-lymph-node metastases. Through interviews with 293 patients, Greenwald et al. (1978) estimated that breast cancer mortality might be reduced by about 19 percent through BSE. A more recent study of 1004 cases by Foster and Costanza (1984) found BSE to be associated with a greater likelihood of detecting one's own cancer, less delay from first symptom to histological diagnosis, earlier clinical stage, smaller pathologic tumor size, fewer axillary node metastases, and perhaps most importantly, significantly increased survival.

In spite of widespread publicity by health promoters, however, the actual rate of BSE practice is surprisingly low. In 1973 the Gallup Organization conducted a national poll at the request of the American Cancer Society and determined that fewer than 25 percent of women ever practice BSE (Gallup Organization, 1973). Stillman (1977) found that 18 percent of a sample of upper middle class women never practiced BSE. Kelly (1979) sampled a highly educated population of women with a breast concern, i.e., all respondents were seeking breast care for breast lumps, breast pain, or other reasons. She determined, that even among a population that one would assume to be conscious of the need for regular BSE, 34 percent of the respondents reported never practicing it. Howe (1981) chose a sample of women who by virtue of sociodemographic characteristics were high risk for breast cancer. She reported that 44 percent of survey respondents reported that they practiced BSE monthly, while 12 percent never practiced it. Turnbull (1978) reported that 22 percent of her respondents, who were women in graduate programs, never practiced BSE. Thus, it is apparent that the rate of BSE practice is variable across samples, but even among relatively high rate samples, the absolute rate is disappointingly low.

There have been some efforts to determine predictors of BSE practice. However, as Reddy (1984) notes, the results of these studies are mixed. For example, Howe (1981) in a sample labeled high-risk for breast cancer, found positive relationships between frequency of BSE practice and the variables of BSE knowledge, BSE attitude, ease of remembering to do BSE, education, and several other factors, but did not find a relationship between perceived cancer risk and frequency of practice. On the other hand, Stillman (1977) did find a relationship between perceived susceptibility to breast cancer and frequency of BSE practice. Kelly (1979) interviewed regular examiners and asked why they originally began practicing BSE. The two most frequent responses were increased awareness that it was important to detect breast cancer early, and increased awareness of the subjects' own personal vulnerability to breast cancer. When the nonexaminer subjects were asked why they did not practice BSE the most frequent response was that for one of a number of reasons (young age, good health, or personal invulnerability) they were not personally at risk for breast cancer. Thus, feelings of personal risk seemed important factors for these subjects in their BSE behavior.

Another way to examine factors associated with BSE practice is to focus not on individual characteristics, but on environmental factors which may facilitate the behavior. This is the tack taken by Grady and her colleagues in a series of studies. For example, Grady, et al. (1982) found that they could increase self-report BSE by rewarding the presentation of completed BSE records with silver dollars. Grady (1984) examined stimulus control of BSE using two methods of cue enhancement: self-managed use of calendars and monthly reminder postcards. She found that postcard reminders worked extremely well in increasing reported BSE practice; however, the timing of the postcards was a crucial variable and, in fact, subjects in the postcard condition who received their postcards at the wrong time were less likely to report BSE practice than subjects who received no postcards at all. The self-management strategy did not have an overall effect. This study also found different results for cyclic or non-cyclic women which suggests that although studying environmental-manipulations that affect BSE may be the direction BSE research is headed, it may still be important to assess subject characteristics which have a direct or indirect affect on compliance with BSE recommendations.

The present study attempted to clarify the psychosocial variables which discriminate regular examiners from non-examiners, to determine the frequency of BSE practice among a college-age population (the age at which monthly practice is recommended to commence), and to determine methods for teaching BSE that appeal to this particular population.

METHOD

In order to clarify the attitudes, behaviors, and background factors associated with BSE, a questionnaire was developed to systematically code subject responses. Results of previous literature were used as a guide in constructing the questionaire. Kelly's (1979) study used an hour-long, in-depth semi-structured interview to obtain responses to questions of interest. The present study asked some of the same questions and used some of the reported responses as options. Other questions and options were added which were either (a) reported in the literature, or (b) of special interest to the experimenter. The final version of the questionnaire was thought to bring together in one instrument questions about many of the possible factors which are related to BSE practice.

Female students enrolled in undergraduate psychology classes completed the survey which was designed to elicit information regarding familiarity with BSE, rate of BSE practice, source of BSE training/information, degree of worry about cancer, knowledge about cure rate of breast cancer, interest in learning more about BSE, and preference for learning setting. Although 325 questionnaires were completed, only those respondents age 20 and over were included in the analyses since 20 is the age at which monthly BSE is recommended to begin. Thus the data from 230 subjects were retained. Depending upon their responses to the question about rate of BSE practice, respondents were directed to answer either (a) a set of questions about their reasons for not practicing BSE and their perception of factors that would increase their likelihood of BSE practice or (b) a set of questions about their reasons for practicing BSE and their reasons for missing a given month's practice. Thus, examiners and nonexaminers answered different questions—only those relevant to them. In addition, all respondents provided some demographic information (age, class, GPA) and information about incidence of breast cancer and other cancers in close relatives.

RESULTS

Age of survey respondents ranged from 20 to 51 with a mean of 23.9 (SD = 6.06). The largest percentage were juniors and seniors (36% and 48% respectively). The mean reported GPA was 2.99 (SD = .56). Twenty-one percent of these respondents reported that a close relative had had breast cancer; 56% reported that a close relative had had cancer other than breast cancer.

On the 230 respondents, 113 were designated as examiners (reporting BSE practice at least 6 times a year). The remaining 117 respondents were classified as non-examiners. Respondents classified as examiners indicated their first, second, and third most important reasons for practicing BSE from a list of six possible responses and an "other" category. The clearly most popular response chosen was "I realize the importance of early detection of breast cancer", which was the first, second, or third choice of 90.3% of the 113 examiner-respondents. The next most popular reason chosen was "My doctor tells me to do it", which was chosen as one of the three main reasons the respondent engaged in BSE by 42.5% of respondents. The other reasons and corresponding percentage of respondents who chose each were "I am confident in my ability to do it correctly" (38.9%), "I am afraid not to do it" (35.4%), "A close friend or relative had breast cancer (34.5%), "It is a habit" (20.4%), and "other" (9.7%).

These examiners-respondents also designated first, second, and third most important reasons for missing BSE practice in a given month from among six listed reasons and an "other" category. The most frequently chosen response was "I forgot" (88.5%). "I was lazy" was chosen as first, second, or third most important reason by 61.9% of respondents. The other reasons and corresponding percentages of respondents who chose each were "It's not necessary to do it every month" (39.8%), "I wasn't confident that I was doing it right" (23%), "I was scared about touching myself" (12.4%), "I was embarrassed about touching myself" (10.6%), and "other" (8.8%).

The 117 respondents who were classified as non-examiners were asked to choose the first, second, and third most important reasons that they did not practice BSE regularly from a list of eight reasons and an "other" category. An overwhelming number of these non-examiner respondents (86.3%) chose "I don't remember to do it" as one of the three most important reasons. Interestingly, the second most often endorsed response was "my health is generally good" which was chosen by 61.5% of these respondents. Forty-six percent endorsed "I don't know how to do it correctly" as one of their reasons for not practicing BSE. Over one-third (38.5%) chose "I would rather not find anything wrong." The remaining reasons and corresponding percentages of respondents who chose them were "It scares me to do it" (16.2%), "It embarrasses me to do it" (12%), "other" (11.1%), "I am too young to need to do it" (7.5%), and "I am not going to get breast cancer" (6%).

These non-examiners were then asked to choose the three occurrences that would render them more likely to practice BSE from a list of eight and an "other" category. Three occurrences were endorsed more than the others and received nearly equal numbers of endorsements. These were "If I was reminded to do it" which was a first, second or third choice of 54.1% of the respondents, "If someone my age I knew well got breast cancer" (58.3%), and "If a family member got breast cancer" (52.1%). The other occurrences and corresponding percentages of respondents who chose them were "If my doctor told me to do it" (45.3%), "If I felt more confident about how to do it right" (41.9%), "If I was informed of the need to detect cancer early" (20.5%), "If I learned how to not be embarrassed by it" (11.1%), "If I was older" (6.8%), and "other" (2.6%).

To distinguish between the 113 examiners and 117 nonexaminers identified by the survey, their responses to the remaining items of the questionnaire were subjected to a stepwise discriminant analysis in order to determine which items successfully differentiated the two groups. The discriminant analysis produced a significant degree of separation between the groups, χ^2 (3) = 90.199, $p < .005$. To interpret the discriminant analysis, standardized discriminant coefficients of the function and the group centroids were examined. The three variables and their corresponding standardized discriminant coefficients were Familiarity with BSE, −.88; Worry about Cancer, −.23; Interest in Learning More About BSE, −.18. Table 1 represents a summary of the analysis.

Thus, the significant predictors of BSE practice among this

TABLE 1

Discriminant Analysis of Examiners vs Non-Examiners

Variable	F to Enter or Remove	Wilks Lambda
Familiarity with BSE	96.13	.7034
Worry About Cancer	7.27	.6816
Want to Learn More about BSE	3.40	.6715

*$p < .005$

sample were familiarity with the technique (more familiarity = greater likelihood of practice), degree of worry about cancer (more worry = greater likelihood of practice), and willingness to learn more about BSE (more willingness = greater likelihood of practice). The examiners obtained a positive centroid loading of .56, which indicates they are most characterized by the above description of the discriminant function. Non-examiners obtained a negative loading of −.58. The obtained discriminant function correctly classified 73.9% of the grouped cases.

Within the total sample, most respondents reported familiarity with BSE. Using a 5-point scale with 1 equal to not at all familiar, and 5 equal to extremely familiar, the mean familiarity rating was 3.8. Only 1.3% of the respondents rated themselves as not at all familiar with BSE, while 63 percent placed themselves in the very or extremely familiar categories. However, in spite of their familiarity with BSE, when asked to categorize themselves in terms of frequency of practice, only 23.5% reported monthly practice. Nearly 15 percent of respondents reported that they never practiced BSE; another 14 percent reported that they practiced it less than once a year.

Respondents were asked to identify where they learned about BSE from among several sources listed on the survey. Physicians were the most frequently cited source (chosen by 35 percent of respondents). The next most frequently cited source (chosen by 27 percent of respondents) was the print media, mostly magazine articles. The remaining 38 percent of responses were distributed among other health professionals (11%), television (6%), mother (5%), friend (2%), and more than one response chosen (14%).

Subjects completed the statement, "If I had the opportunity to learn more about BSE, the likelihood I would take the opportunity is . . . " by using a 5-point Likert Scale with 1 equal to certainly, 2 equal to very likely, 3 equal to possibly, 4 equal to not likely, and 5 equal to certainly not. The mean was 2.28 (SD = .88); the modal response was 2 (very likely), which was chosen by 37% of respondents.

Subjects were asked to designate their preference for further learning about BSE by ranking their first three choices from a list of seven and an "other" category. Female physician was chosen as first, second, or third choice by more respondents than any other response; it was one of the 3 choices of 66% of respondents. Additionally, female nurse was the first, second, and third choice of

62% of respondents. The third most popular choice of settings for learning more about BSE, which was among the 3 choices of 52% of the respondents, was a small group of women similar to the respondent. A private video tape viewing was chosen next most often (by 42% of respondents). Male physician was ranked fifth; only 37% of respondents selected male physician as one of their 3 preferences. Male nurse was chosen by a smaller percentage of respondents than any of the listed choices; this alternative was among the 3 choices of only 10% of respondents.

Using a 5-point scale with 1 equal to not at all, 2 equal to somewhat, 3 equal to moderately, 4 equal to very high, and 5 equal to extremely, respondents rated the degree to which they worry about cancer. The mean response was 2.69 (SD = .91). The modal response was "moderately", chosen by 49% of respondents. When asked to compare the cure rate of breast cancer to that of other cancers, 62% of respondents chose "somewhat higher", 20% chose "about the same" and 9% chose "much higher".

DISCUSSION

The present study provides support for the notion that most college-age women fail to regularly practice BSE, an economical, easily-learned, and efficient detector of breast cancer. Nearly 15 percent of this sample of women college students report that they never practice BSE and another 14 percent report practice less than once a year. Thus, nearly 30 percent of the sample report that they never or rarely engage in BSE practice, in spite of the fact that the American Cancer Society recommends monthly practice by all women age 20 or older. Less than 1 in 4 of this sample report monthly practice.

Because familiarity with BSE was the best discriminator of examiners and non-examiners, it is suggested that this highly effective technique continue to be publicized and promoted. Of course, an interpretation of this finding that cannot be overlooked is that practicing BSE increases one's familiarity with it rather than the other way around. However, making women aware of BSE must be a first step in developing the behavior into a life-long habit.

A distinction can be made between initial exposure to BSE and further learning about the technique. Physicians were cited most often by this college-age sample as a source of initial exposure to

BSE. Although gender was not elicited, based on base rates in the population, it is likely that most of these physicians were male. Ironically, male physicians were ranked fifth among preferred sources for further learning about BSE. Most respondents would choose to learn more about BSE in a person-to-person setting involving another woman or women; the most popular choices were for learning from either a female physician, female nurse, or a small group of similar women. Even viewing a video in private was chosen by a larger percentage of respondents than learning from a male physician. Thus, male physicians might be well advised to have a female nurse or assistant teach BSE technique to their patients.

The second most frequently cited source of initial exposure to BSE was print media, which is probably a reflection of the increased publicity that the technique has gained in recent years. Women's magazines may be appropriate vehicles for introducing BSE, especially to young women. However, after this initial exposure, they may need individual or small group instruction in the technique.

The fact that degree of worry about cancer successfully discriminated examiners from non-examiners, with examiners prone to worry more, presents an interesting dilemma. If one interprets this finding as suggesting that worry increases the likelihood of BSE, then a possible implication is that health promoters should encourage women to worry about cancer, and thereby try to scare them into practicing BSE. However, other studies have concluded that fear and worry may *inhibit* BSE practice (e.g., Gallup, 1973). Further research should clarify the association between BSE and worry. It may be that specific components of worry, such as accurate awareness of personal vulnerability, may facilitate BSE and other components of worry, such as generalized anxiety due to uncertainty, may inhibit the practice. Further support for the notion that the awareness of the personal vulnerability component of worry may promote BSE comes from the finding of the present study that the most popular reason chosen by examiners to explain why they practice BSE was, "I realize the importance of early detection of breast cancer." In order to test the idea that components of worry promote BSE practice, one might develop a package for promoting BSE that combines information about technique with cancer facts designed to make participants aware of (and worried about) their own vulnerability to cancer and to compare the effects on subsequent BSE compliance between this information-worry package and an information only approach to teaching BSE.

An ironic finding of this study is that a significant discriminator of examiners was their interest in learning more about BSE whereas non-examiners were less interested in learning about it. Thus, the women who already practice BSE are the ones who report that they would be likely to take an offered opportunity to learn more about it. This finding suggests that non-examiners may engage in some sort of active denial process about their vulnerability to breast cancer. Further substantiation of this interpretation is the finding that over a third of the non-examiners chose "I'd rather not find anything wrong", as one of their main reasons for not practicing BSE. Additionally, the second most popular choice among non-examiners, chosen by over three-fifths of the sample, was "my health is generally good." This suggests that the non-examiners feel that general good health may protect them from breast cancer.

Several of the findings of this study suggest that women may benefit from reminders to practice BSE. For example, the most common reason chosen by examiners-respondents for missing practice in a given month was that they forgot. Among the non-examiners, the most frequently chosen reason for non-practice was not remembering to do it. Additionally, over half of the non-respondents endorsed "being reminded" as one of the three events that would make them more likely to engage in BSE. Research should continue to focus on the effectiveness of different types of reminders.

In summary, the major findings of this investigation are that: (a) the majority of college women age 20 and over do not practice monthly BSE; (b) women gain initial exposure to BSE from physicians or printed material, but they would choose to learn more about it in a person-to-person setting involving another woman or women; (c) women report that being reminded may increased their BSE compliance (d) there is a positive association between worry about cancer and BSE frequency; and (e) women who already practice BSE are more interested in learning more about it than those who do not.

The findings of this research must be viewed somewhat cautiously as is the case with any study which depends upon self-report. Nonetheless, by their own admission, more than three-quarters of these college women age 20 and older are non-compliant with the American Cancer Society recommendation for monthly breast self-examination. Thus, this study provides base-rate data for a population group which has not previously been studied, and it supports the notion that health care professionals must continue their efforts to involve women in health self-care, specifically BSE.

REFERENCES

American Cancer Society (1986). *1986 Cancer Facts and Figures*. New York: American Cancer Society.

Foster, R.S., Lang, S.P., Costanza, M.C., Worden, J.K., Haines, C.R., & Yates, J.W. (1978). Breast self-examination practices and breast-cancer stage. *N Engl J Med* 299:265–270.

Foster, R.S., & Costanza, M.C. (1984). Breast self-examination practices and breast cancer survival. Cancer 53:167–173.

Gallup Organization, Inc. (1973). *Women's attitudes regarding breast cancer*. New York: Gallup Organization, Inc.

Grady, K.E. (1984). Cue enhancement and the long-term practice of breast self-examination. *J. Behavior Med* 7:191–203.

Grady, K.E., Kegeles, S.S., & Lund, A.K. (1982). Experimental studies to increase BSE—Preliminary findings. *Progr Clin Biol Res* 83:91–105.

Greenwald, P., Nasca, P.C., Lawrence, C.E., Horton, J., McGarrah, R.P., Gabriele, T., & Carlton, K. (1978). Estimated effect of breast self-examination and routine physician examinations on breast-cancer mortality. *N Engl J Med* 299:271–273.

Howe, H.L. (1981). Social factors associated with breast self-examination among high risk women. *Am J Public Health* 71:251–255.

Kelly, P.T. (1979). Breast self-examinations: Who does them and why. *J Behavior Med* 2:31–38.

Reddy, D.M. (1984). Breast self-examination: Correlates and research needs. *The Health Psychologist* 6:3–6.

Silverberg, E., & Lubera, J. (1986). Cancer Statistics, 1986. *CA* 36:9–25.

Stillman, M.J. (1977). Women's health beliefs about breast cancer and breast self-examination. *Nursing Research* 26:121–127.

Turnbull, E.M. (1978). Effect of basic preventive health practice of breast self-examination. *Nursing Research* 27:98–102.

Gender and Illness Behavior Among Colorectal Cancer Patients

James R. Marshall, PhD
Donna P. Funch, PhD

ABSTRACT. This study of 154 men and 152 women with cancer of the colon or rectum addresses the lag between the first recognition of symptoms and the securing of definitive diagnosis and treatment. Total treatment delay is divided into two categories: patient delay, or the lag between the patient's first recognition of symptoms and first physician contact; diagnostic delay, or the lag between the patient's first physician contact and treatment. The results do not support the contention that women are more prone than men to respond to cancer symptoms; women in this sample are not more likely than men to recognize and respond to symptoms and seek care. The results suggest that, among patients with cancer of the rectum, women are more likely than men to delay in seeking care. Among patients with cancer of the colon, women are more likely than men to experience diagnostic delay.

The earlier most cancers are detected, the better the chances of long-term survival or cure (ACS Facts and Figures 1986). Delay in seeking treatment often contributes to late cancer detection. This delay may occur for a variety of reasons. Patients may fail to recognize initially that a symptom is cancer-related or serious enough to deserve professional attention. Once a symptom is recognized, some patients may be reluctant, for a wide range of reasons, to immediately seek care. Finally, there may be variations in the degree to which clinicians regard certain complaints as serious enough to require immediate attention.

It may be useful to consider such practices as seeking and

Reprint requests to James R. Marshall, Department of Social and Preventive Medicine, School of Medicine, State University of New York at Buffalo, 2211 Main Street, Buffalo, NY 14214.

This research was supported, in part, by grant number JFRA-97 from the American Cancer Society.

securing treatment as in large part social. They involve seeking consensual validation from peers regarding whether physical changes or discomfort might be seen as serious symptoms, discussing the need for professional assistance, identifying providers, arranging to be seen, communicating symptoms to clinicians, and complying with recommended procedures.

There are several reasons why it would be useful to assess whether there are substantial differences between men and women in their response to the onset of cancer symptoms, and in their subsequent procurement of diagnosis and treatment. First, survival for some cancers differs by sex, even when stage at diagnosis is considered. Determination of the reasons for these differences may yield clues which will ultimately help improve survival for both sexes. Secondly, many efforts are under way to educate the public on the importance of early detection. These efforts might be better directed if some of the behavioral and motivational differences between men and women were understood.

In addition to describing the process by which people decide that medical care is needed, a study of differences between male and female cancer patients might indicate ways in which cancer control resources could be most efficaciously targeted. If, for example, men were found to recognize symptoms later than women do, it would make sense to try to design programs specifically targeted for men to induce them to respond more promptly to symptoms. If it were discovered that men tend to experience greater lags between physician contact and commencement of treatment, additional resources, including physician education, could be directed toward shortening that lag.

Finally, elucidation of these behavioral differences might help explain some of the differences in survival rates between men and women for certain types of cancer.

Students of health behavior have suggested that men and women respond to different kinds of cues in deciding that medical advice is needed.[1] It is also likely that men and women could seek validation of their symptom perceptions in different ways. It has also been suggested that women and men face different receptions when they appear before a clinician and seek treatment.[2]

Many studies have suggested differences in the sick role behavior of men and women. Davis[3] and Verbrugge,[4] however, have pointed out that a proper understanding of the impact of gender upon illness behavior requires that actual physical condition be taken into account.[3,4] The attribution of gender differences to roles or behavior rather than physical status requires several assumptions regarding the actual physical conditions of the men and women who report different amounts of physical symptoms and engage in different health practices. One method of examining role differences, which would involve minimizing actual physical differences, would be to consider illness behavior for one specific health problem. Colorectal cancer, the second leading cause of cancer-related mortality for both men and women,[5] is especially amenable to this type of study. In a comparison of delay among male and female colorectal cancer patients, disease status could not be a confounding factor.

In one study of delay in treatment-seeking for symptoms in patients with a variety of cancer types, including cancer of the colon, rectum, stomach, lung, leukemia, and lymphoma, two global measures of delay were considered: (1) stage of disease at diagnosis, and (2) the total lag between first notice of symptoms and the recording of a definitive diagnosis.[6] No evidence of differences between men and women were found. While this finding is of interest, a number of limitations restrict the conclusions which can be drawn. First, stage of disease at diagnosis may be affected by a number of factors, including virulence of the specific cancer and genetic predisposition, in addition to illness behavior. An advanced tumor does not necessarily indicate patient delay.

Second, while the lag measure did relate specifically to delay, it focused on the entire interval between detection of the symptoms and diagnosis. This delay interval, however, is composed of several elements. The first of these represents the time between onset and first notice of symptoms. The second period is between the first notice of symptoms and the securing of care, generally labeled in the literature as the patient delay period. During this time, the patient might simply wait to see whether the symptoms persist. He or she might mention them to acquaintances and seek advice as to whether something should be done. The nature of the particular symptoms themselves could affect the duration of this interval. A third possible delay period occurs between first contact with a care provider and the establishment of a diagnosis. A number of factors may result in delay at this stage. Symptoms reported may not suggest cancer to the clinician, or the patient may fail to report the entire constellation of symptoms. The patient may also fail to comply with professional recommendations regarding tests or referrals. In cases such as these, the cancer diagnosis may be delayed until the disease has progressed further. This period of diagnostic delay is generally attributed to the physician, although a number of factors may contribute to its duration.

There is some reason to suspect that each of these phases of delay might be related to gender. For example, women have been described as more health conscious than men;[3] therefore, women may notice symptoms at an earlier point. In addition, women have been described as more willing than men to recognize that they are sick and in need of health care;[1,4] therefore, women who have noticed symptoms may be more likely than men to do something about them. Both factors would seem to contribute to reductions in patient-related delays for women.

On the other hand, the pattern of diagnostic delay might be expected to be somewhat different. It has been suggested that women's problems are treated differently—taken less seriously—than men's problems are.[2] Physicians might be less likely to regard certain symptoms as worrisome if they present in a woman than in a man. Women tend, it has been suggested, to adopt a more deferential role than men do in dealing with health care professionals. Less demanding, they may receive less attention. Vague or poorly defined complaints might be more likely in a woman than in a man to be regarded as idiopathy or as hypochondria. If differential responses on the part of the physician do exist, one would expect to see greater diagnostic delay for women.

As noted earlier, there is a need to examine these issues in samples in which the underlying conditions are known and the symptoms relatively alike for both sexes. This would minimize differences in the physical conditions of men and women.

In this study, gender differences in both patient and diagnostic delay will be considered for a sample of 306 colorectal cancer patients. Information is presented on specific illness behaviors which have been suggested to differ among males and females, including symptom reporting, reactions to symptoms, and perceived barriers to care.

DATA AND METHODS

These data were collected as part of a population-based survey of treatment seeking practices. The study was conducted in the Greater Seattle Metropolitan area between September 1980 and September 1981. Individuals who had been recently diagnosed for colorectal cancer were contacted by telephone and asked to participate in an interview. The interview inquired about the time at which patients had noticed various symptoms of colorectal cancer, any action they took prior to seeking medical treatment, reasons for seeking or waiting to seek treatment in response to these symptoms, and problems encountered in securing care. In total, some 154 male and 152 female cancer patients were interviewed. Of the males, 97 were diagnosed with cancer of the colon, and 55 with cancer of the rectum. Among the females, 109 were diagnosed with cancer of the colon, and 42 with cancer of the rectum. Specific site (colon as opposed to rectum) was not available for 3 cases.

Patients for this study were required to have had a definitive diagnosis (tissue biopsy) of non-recurrent colorectal cancer and to be between the ages of 18 and 85. All patients were resident in King County, Washington. During the one-year period of the study, 521 patients were identified. Of those patients, 28 could not be interviewed because they were deceased, and 31 either spoke no english or would have been unable to provide information because of diagnosed senility. After the case was identified the primary physician, indicated on the registry form, was asked for permission to contact the patient. Physician consent was obtained for 382 patients. Of those, 318 agreed to be interviewed. Twelve of these cases were not included in the analyses presented here, because their responses were judged by the interviewers to be unreliable. The method of data collection and study design are described in more detail elsewhere.[7]

Participants and non participants were compared on major sociodemographic variables: sex, race, marital status, education, stage of disease, and cancer site. None of these differences was statistically significant. Respondents were significantly younger than non respondents, although the magnitude of this difference was small. (~2.6 years).

FINDINGS

Table 1 describes the distribution of study participants by sex and by age, marital status, and education. It can be seen that male patients tended to be younger than female patients. The educational levels of male and female patients tended to be similar. As cancer is a disease of older people, female patients are less likely to be married, and more likely to be widowed, than male patients.

The pattern of symptoms which led respondents to seek care is

Table 1

Characteristics of Colorectal Cancer Study Respondents [1]

	MALE (n=154) #	MALE (n=154) %	FEMALE (n=152) #	FEMALE (n=152) %
Age				
60	29	19	40	26
60-69	61	39	39	26
70-79	43	28	56	37
80+	21	14	17	11
Education (Grade Completed)				
1-8	22	14	18	12
9-11	24	16	24	16
12	45	29	58	38
13-16	44	29	42	28
17+	18	12	10	6
Marital Status				
Single	8	5	5	3
Married	125	81	80	53
Widowed	13	8	47	31
Separated/Divorced	8	5	20	13

[1] Numbers may vary slightly due to missing information.

described in detail in Table 2. Since the symptom constellations of patients with cancer of the colon and of the rectum were generally similar, the sites are grouped. The percentages of male and female patients reporting each symptom are presented in the upper portion of the table. The most common symptom for both males and females is bleeding; general weakness and abdominal pain were also quite common. The proportions of male and female patients reporting any one prediagnostic symptom are not significantly different. The total number of symptoms reported is also considered but the difference is not significant.

While these findings suggest that symptom reporting is generally similar for men and women in this study, it is possible that there could be gender differences in the intensity of those symptoms.

Table 2

Prediagnostic Symptoms of Colorectal Cancer Patients

Individual Symptoms Experienced	Male n=152 %	Female n=149 %	
Constipation	34	33	
Diarrhea	24	30	
Bleeding	64	65	
Gas	44	51	
Mucus in Stool	13	17	
Bowel Evacuation Problem	22	20	
Abdominal Pain	41	46	
Rectal Pain	8	7	
Appetite Loss	23	21	
Weight Loss	29	22	
Weakness	51	60	
	Mean Male (sd)	Mean Female (sd)	t-value (significance)
Total Number of Symptoms Reported	3.5 (2.0)	3.7 (2.0)	1.13 (n.s.)
Severity of Symptoms (1 to 3 with 3 indicating very severe)	1.5 (0.8)	1.4 (0.8)	-.66 (n.s.)
Percentage of Symptoms Developing Slowly	31% (30.9)	33% (32.7)	.63 (n.s.)
Percentage of Symptoms With Rapid Onset	22% (30.1)	15% (25.1)	-1.93 (.06)

Not Significant ($P < .10$)

Some specific information on each of the reported symptoms was available and in presented in the bottom half of Table 2. For example, subjects were asked to rate the severity of any symptom experienced and a mean severity score was computed. There is essentially no difference between males and females in assessed severity of symptoms. Subjects were also asked to categorize the rapidity with which these symptoms developed (rapid onset, slow onset, or other). The mean percentages of symptoms developing slowly or rapidly for males and females are presented in Table 2. Both men and women report approximately one-third of their symptoms as developing slowly. Male patients are more likely to report that symptoms developed quickly although the difference between males and females is of only marginal significance. Overall, these findings suggest that, for colorectal cancer patients, males and females report the same symptoms and describe them in a similar manner.

Even if symptom perceptions of males and females are similar, there may be differences in the way in which males and females respond to these symptoms. Table 3 describes mean *patient* delay. This delay is operationalized as the lag in days between the date of the first notice of symptoms and the date when the subject first contacted a physician for treatment of those symptoms. If both colon and rectal cancers are grouped together, the difference be-

Table 3

Mean Patient Delay in Days, Males and Females

Colorectal Cancer Patients

		MALE	FEMALE	t-value (significance)
Total	Mean	180.0	198.7	.73
	(sd)	(214.9)	(220.2)	(n.s.)
Colon	Mean	198.4	179.5	-.59
	(sd)	(228.0)	(213.0)	(n.s.)
Rectum	Mean	149.3	254.9	2.37
	(sd)	(191.1)	(233.5)	(.02)

tween male and female patients in delay is not statistically significant, although female patients tend to delay about 10 percent longer than male patients. Patient delay, however, is composed of two distinct patterns which appear to differ substantially. Among colon cancer patients, males tend to delay slightly longer. This difference is far from statistically significant. On the other hand, among patients with cancer of the rectum, female patients delay, on average, considerably longer. This difference of approximately 100 days is statistically significant. To assess the extent to which this difference was the result of outliers (extreme values) in the data, a logarithmic transformation, comparing mean male and female delay in logarithms, was utilized. The results of these analyses were essentially the same as those presented in Table 3.

Patients in this study were questioned on reasons for delaying in seeking care. Because of the substantial male-female difference in rectal cancer delay, the data were examined to determine what role various problems might play in the excess delay for female patients. These include problems with transportation, getting time off from work, not knowing where to go for help, not thinking the disease was serious, discomfort with physicians, fear, the belief that physicians can't help, and being too busy. A summary index composed of the respondent's total number of reported problems or barriers was also used. The extent to which each of these problems was reported by males and females is presented in Table 4. There were no significant differences in reported problems related to delay, and adjustment for these did not alter the association between gender and patient delay. Differences in patient delay persisted with adjustment for age and education.

Other aspects of treatment seeking could be related to this male-female difference. These could include the numbers of people with whom symptoms were discussed, self-medication by the use of over-the-counter drugs, and reading about symptoms before seeing a doctor. Male-female differences in these behaviors are presented in Table 5. It can be seen that the percentages of men and women reading about their symptoms are not significantly different. Men and women took similar numbers of over-the-counter drugs, and talked to similar numbers of people about their symptoms. The percentages of men and women discussing their symptoms with spouse or friends were not significantly different. Women were significantly more likely to discuss their symptoms with children

Table 4

Male, Female Differences: Problems Causing Rectal Cancer Patient Delay

Problem	% Reporting Male	Female
Transportation Problem	4	7
Problem Getting Time Off	9	12
Didn't Know Where to Go for Help	9	8
Not Serious	62	54
Discomfort With Doctors	22	11
Fear	22	15
Thought Doctor Couldn't Help	8	5
Was Too Busy	19	22
Total Number of Problems (Mean)	1.18	1.20
(sd)	(.17)	(.18)

and with other relatives. Adjustment for these, however, did not diminish the male-female difference.

Diagnostic delay, operationally defined as the lag in days between the patient's first call or visit and definitive diagnosis, is addressed in Table 6. It can be seen that there is a substantial difference in diagnostic delay experienced by males and females for both sites combined. A separate examination of each site revealed that this difference was due entirely to the greater diagnostic delay experienced by women with colon cancer.

A number of characteristics of males and females could conceivably have a bearing on the difference in their diagnostic delay. The respondent's having received some urging from acquaintances that medical services were warranted could be related to diagnostic delay. A patient whose significant others are strongly urging him or her to seek treatment might be more demanding and receive a more prompt diagnosis. The differences between men and women in talking with others about their symptoms are considered in Table 7. It can be seen that both men and women are likely to discuss their symptoms with their spouse. As with rectal cancer, women tend to be more likely to discuss symptoms with their children and are significantly more likely than men to discuss their problems with other relatives. Adjustment for these differences, however, did not substantially alter the male-female difference in diagnostic delay. Patient delay was also considered. Diagnostic delay could clearly be negatively related to patient delay; diagnostic delay could be expected to be very short if patient delay had been long. Adjustment for patient delay, together with age and education, did not eliminate or greatly lessen the male-female difference in delay. The difference between males and females remains statistically significant.

Separate analyses revealed that the number of physician visits before diagnosis is related to the length of physician delay. Thus, women who had longer total physician delays also reported that they had visited the doctor more times before a diagnosis was reached. With the number of visits before diagnosis held constant, the difference between males and females is diminished to the point of statistical insignificance. This suggests that a substantial proportion of the male-female difference in physician delay is a function of the

Table 5

Response Activities of Male and Female Rectal Cancer Patients to Symptoms

Activity	Male	Female	Significance
Reading About Symptoms (%)	10	16	n.s.
Number of Over-the-Counter Drugs Taken to Relieve Symptoms [Mean, (sd)]	1.29 (1.27)	1.26 (0.83)	n.s.
Number of People With Whom Symptoms Discussed [Mean, (sd)]	1.25 (0.90)	1.55 (1.36)	n.s.
Percent Discussing Symptoms With:			
Spouse	76	68	n.s.
Children	17	50	.004
Other Relatives	13	28	.03
Friends	31	38	n.s.

Table 6

Mean Diagnostic Delay in Days, Male vs. Female Cancer Patients

	Male	(sd)	Female	(sd)	t-value (significance)
Total	67.0	(104.7)	106.1	(175.0)	2.35 (.02)
Colon	71.7	(101.1)	125.7	(197.5)	2.49 (.01)
Rectum	59.4	(112.8)	56.5	(79.4)	-.15 (n.s.)

Table 7

Differences Between Male and Female Colon Cancer Patients in Discussing Symptoms With Others*

Percent Respondents Discussing Symptoms With:	Male %	Female %	Chi-Square (1 d.f.)	P
Spouse	80	68	2.20	n.s.
Children	26	42	3.46	.06
Other Relatives	11	30	8.59	.003
Friends	33	42	1.48	n.s.
Total No. Consulted (Mean)	1.38	1.54	t=.95	n.s.
(sd)	(1.08)	(1.18)		

*Percentages are calculated on basis of number of people who have that source available.

excess in physicican visits by female patients before the physician arrived at a diagnosis. The exact reason for excess number of visits is not known. Patients did provide some data on the reason for each of the delays experienced during the treatment-seeking process, with delays defined as periods exceeding 14 days between contacts with health professionals. These reasons were categorized into those due to scheduling problems (office or laboratory), physician-related (e.g., misdiagnosis, "watching and waiting"), or patient-related (e.g., cancelling follow-up visit, deciding to monitor symptoms). Detailed information on the classification of these delays is available elsewhere.[7]

The percentages of males and females reporting each of these reasons for diagnostic delay are provided in Table 8. No difference in scheduling delay was reported, while there was a tendency for women to experience more physician-related delays. Of particular interest is the significantly larger numbers of patient-related delays for women during the diagnostic interval. This suggests that women may contribute to the delay in diagnosis themselves by practices which may defer diagnosis. It is also possible that women are more willing to report this type of behavior than men.

DISCUSSION

The analysis provides little support to the common claim that women are more likely than men to respond to symptoms of illness by seeking medical care. Female colorectal cancer patients did not, according to these observations, report with disease at earlier stages than those at which male colorectal cancer patients reported. Female

Table 8

Reasons for Diagnostic Delay: Colon Cancer

Reason[a]	% Reporting Male (n=95)	Female (n=107)	Chi-Square (1 d.f.)	P
Scheduling Problems	20	15	.56	n.s.
Physician-Related	21	32	2.45	.11
Patient-Related	10	22	4.30	.04

[a]See text and reference 7 for detailed definitions.

colorectal cancer patients did not delay less than male patients in seeking medical care; for rectal cancer they tended to delay longer. They also experienced more delay than men securing definitive diagnosis subsequent to having consulted a clinician.

The degree to which these findings may be generalized to all disease or cancer behaviors should not be overstated. Indeed, the data suggest that differences between men and women in the process of seeking medical care depend heavily on the site of the cancer. The patterns of delay observed appear to be different for cancers of the colon than for those of the rectum.

There has been considerable debate over the extent to which illness behavior differences between men and women reflect a pervasive pattern which would apply to all health behavior.[4,8,9] These results, which suggest that male-female differences depend on whether the site is the colon or the rectum, provide little support to Gove and Hughes' contention that a parsimonious explanation of sick role differences could be applied to conditions as diverse as mental disorder and chronic disease.[9]

There are slight differences in the symptom patterns presented by cancer of the colon as opposed to cancer of the rectum.[10] Cancer of the rectum, in general, produces more vivid and obvious symptoms, so is slightly more likely than cancer of the colon to be discovered at an early stage. This is particularly true for bleeding, which is reported in about 80 percent of all rectal cancer diagnoses, but in only about 50 percent of colon cancer diagnoses. Whether differences in the symptomatology of these conditions could be responsible for the specificity of delay differences deserves more study.

One of the motivations of this paper was to examine the possibility that social roles—those linked to sex—might have some bearing on the process of illness identification and response. We noticed, however, that there were few differences between males and females for many of the illness behaviors that have been postulated to differ between males and females. Thus, symptom reporting, the extent of perceived problems of access and perceived barriers to care, as well as health reporting behavior, did not appear to be greatly different among male and female patients who had similar kinds of diseases.

A troubling result of this study is the observation that, among patients with cancer of the colon, diagnostic delay appears to be much greater for women than for men. This delay difference is not apparent for patients with cancer of the rectum. We are not certain why this result would apply only to patients with cancer of the colon, although rectal cancers may be more readily detected by physicians by virtue of their location and presenting symptoms.

SUMMARY

Among patients with cancer of the colon, symptoms are more likely to be ill-defined, vague, and diffuse than those of patients with cancer of the rectum. Pain may be less acute. If symptoms are poorly defined, physicians may interpret those symptoms differently among women than among men. These possibilities deserve additional investigation. The excess delay could be an artifact of small numbers. The numbers of male and female patients with cancer of the colon and of the rectum in this study, however, are large enough that the differences observed would be very unlikely to occur by chance: The delay differences observed here would be unlikely unless there were some true difference in diagnostic delay accorded male and female colon cancer patients. If this difference is not artifactual, then increased clinical attention to such vague complaints and symptoms as may be indicative of incipient colorectal cancer among women may be warranted. These data, which suggest more substantial delay among female than among male patients, may indicate that symptoms of these two cancers are overlooked as a function of the sex of the person presenting the symptoms.

One problem with empirical data is that they are often inconsiderate of elaborate hypotheses and theoretical constructs. In this study of men and women with colorectal cancer, we found, contrary to a substantial body of theoretical expectation, that women are not more prone than men to seek treatment for intensifying disease symptoms. They tend to delay longer than men in responding to symptoms. Second, we found that men and women do not appear to differ on a number of behaviors that have been advanced as explanations of women's greater willingness to respond to symptoms. Finally, we found that, among colon cancer patients, women encounter greater diagnostic delay than men do. Part of this delay could be attributed to factors for which the patient was responsible. Part of it seemed to be a function of female patients' needing more appointments before a diagnosis was produced. It remains a possibility that clinicians respond differently to women than to men when confronted with the diffuse and poorly defined symptoms of colon cancer.

NOTES

1. Mechanic, D. (1977). Sex, Illness Behavior and the Use of Health Services. *Journal of Human Stress*, 2:29–40.

2. Nathanson, C. (1977). Sex, Illness and Medical Care: A Review of Data, Theory and Method. *Social Science and Medicine*, 11:13–25.

3. Davis, M. (1981). Sex Differences in Reporting Osteoarthritic Symptoms: A Sociomedical Approach. *Journal of Health and Social Behavior*, 22:298–309.

4. Verbrugge, L.M. (1985). Gender and Health: An Update of Hypotheses and Evidence. *Journal of Health and Social Behavior*, 26:156–182.

5. Silverberg, E. (1985). Cancer Statistics, 1985. *Ca-A Cancer Journal for Clinicians*, 35th 1:19–35.

6. Marshall, J.R., Gregorio, D.I., & Walsh, D. (1982). Sex Differences in Illness Behavior: Care Seeking Among Cancer Patients. *Journal of Health and Social Behavior*, 23:197–204.

7. Funch, D.P. (1985). Diagnostic Delay in Symptomatic Colorectal Cancer. *Cancer*, 56:2120–2124.

8. Mechanic, D. (1980). Comment on Gove and Hughes. *American Sociological Review*, 45:513–514.

9. Gove, W., & Hughes, M. (1979). Possible Causes of the Apparent Sex Differences in Health: An Empirical Investigation. *American Sociological Review*, 45:514–522.

10. Schwartz, S.I. (1969). *Principles of Surgery*. McGraw-Hill Book Company, New York.

Women and Preventive Health Care: An Exploratory Study of the Use of Pap Smears in a Potentially High-Risk Appalachian Population

Sue Fisher, PhD
Ann L. Page, PhD

ABSTRACT. In the United States, medical services are organized to provide acute and chronic care. In such a system, people may not receive the routine preventive care necessary for the maintenance of their health. This study, conducted in the model family practice clinic of a residency training program, reports on the use of a preventive health measure (i.e., Pap smears) in a potentially high-risk population. The odds of receiving the Pap smear were calculated for selected variables for 253 patients. The most important variables for distinguishing the outcome (Pap/no Pap) were age and the medical reason for the visit. Although there was some indication that high-risk women were targeted for screening, our findings most strongly supported the claim that Pap smears were performed in this setting when they were requested, required, or convenient.

Today the delivery of medical care is one of the most crucial problems facing our society. There is a growing concern with the quality and availability of medical care as well as with the escalation of medical costs. One consequence of this dissatisfaction is that health care and prevention are becoming critical issues in the 1980s. However, prevention is at odds with the structure of our current medical system and therefore is only nominally dealt with in the medical training process.

Sue Fisher is an Assistant Professor of Sociology and the Science in Society Program at Wesleyan University, Middletown, CT 06457. Ann L. Page is an Associate Professor of Sociology at Appalachian State University, Boone, NC 28608.

We recognize that the organization of a medical care system is not without health consequences. A distinction can be made between a system organized to provide medical care (i.e., a medical care system for the diagnosis and treatment of illness) and one oriented toward maintaining the health of the population by preventing illness (i.e., a health care system). Critics (Knowles, 1977; Sidel & Sidel in Conrad & Kern, 1981; Taylor, 1982; Terris, 1980) contend that in the United States we have a far greater investment in the treatment rather than in the prevention of illness. In general, our medical care system is organized to provide acute, curative, and chronic care and is becoming increasingly hospital-centered and dependent on expensive high technology. Lip service is paid to the virtues of preventive health care but the monies allocated for this purpose are low and, with current trends, getting lower. This is the case despite the fact that epidemiological findings support the use of preventive measures to assure savings in terms of illness, lives, and medical costs (Taylor, 1982; Terris, 1980).

In a medical care system oriented toward treatment, people may not receive the routine preventive care necessary for the maintenance of their health. This study reports on the use of a preventive measure (i.e., Pap smears)[1] in a potentially high-risk population—Appalachian women. The research was conducted at a model family practice clinic affiliated with a teaching hospital in the southeastern part of the United States. The clinic provided an ideal research setting to investigate the performance of this procedure since Family Medicine, as a primary care specialty, is assumed to have a strong orientation toward preventive care. If we are to find a commitment to prevention among medical providers, we would expect to find it among these physicians.

PAP SMEAR SCREENING AND CERVICAL CANCER

Approximately 6,800 women are expected to die in this country in 1986 from cervical cancer. Because this disease is often without symptoms in the early stages, the use of a preventive health measure (i.e., Pap smears) is especially important (American Cancer Society, 1986).[2] Accepted as a reliable and practical diagnostic technique, the Pap smear procedure increases the opportunity to identify potential disease, maximizes the likelihood of early treatment, and minimizes the potential of mortality from cervical cancer. Numerous studies have shown that comprehensive cytological screening programs increase early detection and therefore decrease mortality from the disease (Boyes, 1972; Boyes et al., 1977; Brown, 1976; Burns et al., 1968; Cramer, 1974; Dickinson et al., 1972; Handy & Wieben, 1965; Lundin et al., 1965; Lynge, 1983; Sall et al., 1968; Timonen et al., 1974; Walton et al., 1979). Direct correlations have been demonstrated between the intensity of the screening program and reduction of this cancer (Boyes et al., 1977; Draper & Cook, 1983). Such reductions were achieved through screening and early treatment of precancerous conditions (Christopherson et al., 1970; Lundin et al., 1965). While recent studies have suggested that yearly Pap smears are not needed for all populations of women, no suggestion has been made to discontinue them. Instead, the populations most likely to benefit have been pinpointed. A strong case is made for encouraging a consistent Pap smear screening program as a routine feature of medical examinations, especially in high-risk populations (Marx, 1979; Shulman et al., 1974).

Studies suggest that a constellation of factors is prominent among women who develop cervical cancer. The age factor is an important variable in a study by Marshall (1965). The mean age at the time of discovery was 40.7 years for pre-invasive cancer and 50.3 years for invasive cancer. Furthermore, a profile developed by Walton and colleagues (1979) suggests that women with cervical cancer are more often lower socioeconomic class, rural, and with long intervals since their last pregnancy. In a similar study, Handy and Wieben (1965) focus on a socioeconomic complex of relative poverty, rapid sexual maturation, and haste—the early beginning and early termination of the reproductive phase. In addition, the incidence of cervical cancer was significantly higher among the Blacks in their study than the whites, and within the white group, higher among lower income categories. They suggest that sexual maturation, intercourse, and pregnancy occur significantly earlier in the lives of women who develop this cancer and that age at first coitus, number of sex partners, and penile hygiene may also explain some of the variance in incidence for different populations (e.g., Black/white, urban/rural, higher/lower social class) (see also Graham & Schotz, 1979).

There is some indication from these studies that the women who would benefit most from a comprehensive screening program for cervical cancer are not being routinely examined. A two year study (Walton et al., 1979) of patients with advanced carcinoma of the cervix found that only 12 percent had the disease diagnosed by a screening examination before the onset of symptoms. Furthermore, 36 percent of the women were not diagnosed even though they had been exposed to the medical care system. Another study by Fruchter et al. (1980) reports on the health care history of women with invasive cervical cancer. Fifty-two percent had no previous Pap smears and 62 percent had no Pap smears during the preceding five year period. However, 73 percent of the unscreened women had received ambulatory medical care, including 41 percent who had regular care for chronic conditions and 16 percent who had been hospitalized. The Walton et al. study (1979) and another by Marshall (1965) suggest that sexually active, lower socioeconomic women past their primary reproductive years are often out of the mainstream of the medical care system where they would be more likely to receive routine Pap smears (e.g., during examinations for birth control methods, during pre- and post-natal care, as a feature of venereal disease screening, or while being treated for vaginal infections). Similarly, Fruchter and colleagues (1980) conclude that much of the low income population could be reached by routine screening in ambulatory health services and hospitals.

Although the importance of Pap smears as a preventive measure has been clearly established, opinion is divided as to who is responsible for initiating the necessary screening. One view places the responsibility with the physician. The claim is that the management of pre-invasive cervical lesions is so effective that "physicians should offer Pap smears to all patients regardless of presenting complaint" (*Ob, Gyn News*, 1983). The other view places the responsibility with the patient. For example, a reproductive oncologist in the region where this study was conducted expresses the opinion that a great many women in this area are "ignoring their gynecological health by avoiding annual physicals and such easy diagnostic tests as Pap smears" (Veal, 1983). Unfortunately, many women anticipate or experience pelvic examinations and Pap smears as uncomfortable, anxiety-producing, often degrading procedures (Emerson in Dreitzel, 1970; Knopf, 1976; Magee, 1975). Furthermore, the preventive implications of these techniques are not always well understood by patients (Knopf, 1976). Since cervical examinations are generally performed in doctors' offices and women are usually introduced to Pap smears by their physicians, doctors clearly play the most important role in influencing patients to have these procedures (Burns et al., 1968; Kegeles, 1967; McCurtis, 1979; Walton et al., 1979). It is apparent that the routine performance of

Pap smears and the success of cytological screening programs depend to a large extent on the interest, knowledge, and cooperation of medical providers (Kegeles, 1967).

In view of these previous studies, the model family practice clinic described here seemed to offer a useful setting to explore the performance of Pap smears. The residents in this program are being trained to provide primary care, often in rural, mountain communities in the region.[3] The patient population that they will treat is by definition potentially at high risk. Appalachian women are at risk for several reasons. First, the region has the highest rate of cervical cancer in the United States (Kleinman, 1979; Mason & McKay, 1969). Second, the Appalachian region is a poverty area and as such has a large population of women who have a high potential for developing disease and a low utilization of medical services. Third, Appalachia is a medically underserved area (Fowinkle, 1975).[4] One characteristic of such areas is that, for the most part, medical care is provided by primary care physicians such as the doctors under study in our case. These providers are assumed to share a commitment to care for the whole person in the context of their daily lives (Flannery, 1982). This assumption underlies the belief that family practitioners have a stronger orientation toward primary care and prevention than is typically the case for those practicing in other medical specialties.

The purpose of this research is to describe the characteristics of patients who receive a Pap smear during visits to this clinic in comparison to patients who do not. Such information could be especially useful because a large proportion of the primary care physicians who practice in Appalachia are trained in medical schools and residency programs in the area.

METHOD

Sample

As mentioned above, the data reported in this paper were collected at a university medical center. Specifically, the research setting was the center's family practice residency training program. This program was designed to model a fee-for-service practice in Family Medicine. Residents in the three year program provided primary care to patients.[5] Emergency procedures were usually performed elsewhere and those who needed specialized care were generally referred.

Data were collected (from personal file questionnaires which new patients complete and from medical records) for all female patients (aged 14 and over) who came to the family practice program for the first time between June 15, 1981 and October 31, 1981. Data collection continued for each patient for three visits, until a program resident performed a Pap smear or until June 1, 1982, whichever came first.

The analysis presented below focuses on the visit data from medical records together with selected data from the patients' file questionnaires. Due to their secondary nature, the variables were necessarily limited in number and type. Additional information obtained from observations at the center is used in the concluding section to aid in the interpretation of the findings.

Measures

Sociodemographic Variables. Four of the patient background measures were coded as dummy variables: (1) marital status (married/not married), (2) race (white/non-white), (3) student status (student/non-student), and (4) employment status (employed/not employed). Age was measured in years at time of visit. The coding categories for education and income were taken from the patient file questionnaire. Education completed and income were coded into five and eight categories respectively. Type of insurance was interpreted as a measure of ability to pay and was coded as: (1) none, (2) public, and (3) private. Public insurance was defined as medical payments from public funds (e.g., Medicaid or Medicare), while private insurance involved payments from private companies via group or individual policies.

Visit Variables. There were six visit variables derived from patient medical records. Year of residency of examining doctor and number of visit were coded first, second, or third. The medical reason for the visit was coded as: (1) general physical, (2) pelvic indicator, or (3) nonpelvic complaint. A general physical was indicated if the patient requested a physical, had a chronic condition (e.g., hypertension, diabetes) where a physical was necessary to assess general health status, or had a range of non-specific symptoms which suggested various diagnoses. Pelvic indicator was coded as the reason for the visit if the patient requested a Pap smear, requested a birth control method, or had a specific medical condition which would place the doctor in the pelvic area to reach a diagnosis (e.g., pregnancy, vaginal infection, vaginal bleeding, painful intercourse, or pain in lower right or left quadrant of the abdomen). Nonpelvic complaint was indicated if the patient had a specific complaint that would not place the doctor in the pelvic area (e.g., sore throat). The final visit measure was coded as a dummy variable for performance of a Pap smear (Pap/no Pap).

Analysis

Frequency distributions for each variable by age category were constructed for each visit. These distributions were then crosstabulated with the outcome variable (Pap/noPap). Further analysis was conducted on the first visit data only. Cell frequencies for second and third visit data were too small to warrant further consideration.

For first visit patients, the odds ratio for receiving a Pap smear was estimated for each category of each variable with one of the values being chosen as a reference category. Ratios also were calculated for each variable controlling for age. The odds ratio is a measure of association which compares the risk of experiencing the outcome under study (Pap/no Pap) when an antecedent factor is present with the risk the outcome will occur when the antecedent is absent (Fleiss, 1981).

RESULTS

The mean age of the patients at first visit (N = 253) was 33.2 years. Fifty-five percent were married and 87 percent were white. Fifty-five percent were employed, while 12 percent were students. Twenty-two percent had no insurance, 22 percent had public insurance, and 56 percent had private coverage. Nineteen percent had 8 or fewer years of education, 51 percent had 9–12 years, and 30 percent had more than 12 years. Forty-five percent of the patients had incomes of $8,000 or less, 37 percent had $8,001–$15,000, 8 percent had $15,001–$21,000, and 9 percent had $21,001 or above. On the visit variables, 5.5 percent saw a first year resident, 43.5 percent a second year resident, and 51 percent a third year resident. The distribution of patients on the medical reason for first visit variable was 17.4 percent for general physical, 30 percent for pelvic indicator, and 52.6 percent for nonpelvic complaint.

While four of the variables mentioned above (marital status, race, student status, year of residency) showed no significant change in distribution over the three visit period, the findings do indicate several interesting patterns by visit. First, the percentage of patients in the first four age categories (<20, 20–29, 30–39, 40–49) declined with each visit but increased in the 50 and above age group (15.4 percent-28.8 percent-31.4 percent). We assume that this pattern is due to older women having more medical problems. A second pattern is apparent in the medical reason for visit variable. The percentage of patients in the general physical (17.4 percent-10.6 percent-7.8 percent) and pelvic indicator (30 percent-26 percent-17.6 percent) categories declined with each visit, while the nonpelvic complaint category (52.6 percent-63.5 percent-74.5 percent) showed an increase. This may be due to the fact that "nonpelvic complaint" represented a much more general category than the other two classifications. A third pattern by visit is of special interest for this study. Four variables which possibly reflect socioeconomic status showed an increasing percentage of lower status patients with each visit. There was a higher percentage of patients with public insurance (21.7 percent-28.8 percent-39.2 percent) with each visit. The percentage of patients with 8 years or less of education increased (18.7 percent-28.1 percent-31.3 percent) as did the lowest income category (45 percent-51.6 percent-52.1 percent). The percentage of unemployed patients also increased (45 percent-49.5 percent-58.3 percent) with each visit. We are especially interested in this pattern since lower socioeconomic status women are a high-risk group for cervical cancer.

The distribution for the outcome variable showed that 77 (30 percent) of the 253 first visit patients received a Pap smear, while 176 (70 percent) did not. Of the 176 who did not, 104 (59 percent) returned for a second visit. On the second visit, 20 (19 percent) received a Pap smear and 84 (81 percent) did not. Of those 84, 51 (61 percent) returned for a third visit. Four (8 percent) received a Pap smear and 47 (92 percent) did not. There was a mean of 6.1 weeks between visits one and two. Between visits two and three, there was a mean of 8.1 weeks.

Notably, if a Pap smear was not done on the first visit, it was less likely to be done on later visits (30 percent-19 percent-8 percent). This was the case *regardless* of the reason for visit. The pattern was especially evident for the pelvic indicator category (74 percent-52 percent-33 percent). For the general physical (29.5 percent-27.3

percent-22 percent) and nonpelvic complaint (6 percent-4.5 percent-0 percent) categories, the pattern existed but was less strong. The implications of this finding will be discussed in the conclusion.

Table 1 shows the odds ratio of receiving a Pap smear for each

TABLE I.

Odds Ratios of Receiving a Pap Smear for 253 First Visit Women by Selected Variables

	Pap		No Pap		
	(N)	(%)	(N)	(%)	Odds Ratio
Age					
50 and above	4	(5%)	35	(20%)	1.0*
40-49	10	(13%)	13	(7%)	6.7
30-39	14	(18%)	39	(22%)	3.1
20-29	28	(36%)	71	(40%)	3.5
Less than 20	21	(27%)	18	(10%)	10.3
Total	77		176		
Insurance					
Public	14	(18%)	41	(23%)	1.0*
Private	43	(56%)	98	(56%)	1.3
None	20	(26%)	37	(21%)	1.6
Total	77		176		
Marital status					
Not married	30	(41%)	76	(47%)	1.0*
Married	44	(59%)	84	(53%)	1.3
Total	74		160		
Race					
White	63	(86%)	140	(88%)	1.0*
Not white	10	(14%)	19	(12%)	1.2
Total	73		159		
Education					
0 - 8 years	11	(15%)	32	(20%)	1.0*
9 - 12 years	43	(59%)	75	(48%)	1.7
College and above	19	(26%)	50	(32%)	1.1
Total	73		157		
Student status					
Not student	61	(84%)	141	(90%)	1.0*
Student	12	(16%)	16	(10%)	1.4
Total	73		157		

TABLE 1 (continued)

Employment status					
Employed	36	(49%)	91	(58%)	1.0*
Not employed	37	(51%)	67	(42%)	1.4
Total	73		158		
Income					
Less than $8000	30	(42%)	71	(46%)	1.0*
$8000 - $15000	28	(39%)	56	(36%)	1.2
$15001 - $21000	6	(8%)	13	(8%)	1.1
$21001 and above	7	(10%)	14	(9%)	1.2
Total	71		154		
Year of residency					
Third year	29	(38%)	100	(57%)	1.0*
Second year	44	(57%)	66	(37%)	2.3
First year	4	(5%)	10	(6%)	1.4
Total	77		176		
Medical reason for visit					
Nonpelvic complaint	8	(10%)	125	(71%)	1.0*
General physical	13	(17%)	31	(18%)	6.5
Pelvic indicator	56	(73%)	20	(11%)	43.7
Total	77		176		

Total figures vary becuase of missing values.

* Reference population.

category of each variable (visit one only). Using these odds ratios, it is possible to construct a descriptive profile of the Pap patient group. In comparison to patients who did not receive a Pap smear, Pap patients in this study were disproportionately: under 20 years of age (odds ratio = 10.3) or between 40 and 49 years (odds ratio = 6.7), had no insurance (odds ratio = 1.6), were married (odds ratio = 1.3), non-white (odds ratio = 1.2), had 9–12 years of education (odds ratio = 1.7), were students (odds ratio = 1.7), were not employed (odds ratio = 1.4), saw a second year resident (odds ratio = 2.3), and had a pelvic indicator as the medical reason for visit (odds ratio = 43.7). However, as the table shows, some of these relationships were relatively weak. The strongest variables for distinguishing the outcome (Pap/no Pap) were age and medical reason for visit.

When age was controlled, four of the Pap group profile characteristics (insurance, marital status, race, education) described above were no longer evident. Among the remaining variables, the student status relationship was still apparent but declined with age to zero. Women who were not employed were more likely to receive a Pap smear until the 50 and above age group. The pattern of second year residents doing more Pap smears generally held across age categories. The strongest variable for distinguishing the outcome when age was controlled was still medical reason for visit. Overall, the odds for receiving a Pap smear were highest in the under 20 and 40–49 age categories for all of the variables, indicating that age was a significant determinant of the outcome. The relationship between these two age categories and the risks associated with cervical cancer will be discussed in the conclusion.

CONCLUSION

Initially, the model family practice clinic described in this study appeared to be a setting conducive to the routine performance of Pap smears. The clinic was a teaching situation, without either the economic motives (i.e., the residents and attending staff were salaried) or the extreme time pressures normally associated with a private fee-for-service medical practice. However, we found that of the 253 first visit patients, only 41.5 percent received a Pap smear during the study period. Whether this screening rate is high or low is problematic. We would suggest that it is low considering the setting and the high-risk Appalachian population.[6] The philosophy of primary care implies that family practitioners are the first line of defense in patient health care. This expectation was especially important for our study setting because of the nature of the population served. Because the region is characterized by a low utilization of medical services, *each* patient visit is important. If women do not receive Pap smears on such visits, studies (e.g., Burns et al., 1968; Kegeles, 1967) have shown that they are not likely to return for tests or for other preventive procedures.

We were also concerned to find that if Pap smears were not done on first visits, they were less likely to be done on subsequent visits. This was the case regardless of the medical reason for the visit. In private practice, this finding might reflect the physician's general concern with time. If time were a problem, we would expect that if doctors did not ask a question or do a procedure on one visit, it might be done on a later visit. However, the residents in this study were under no such time pressures. Neither can we explain this finding by claiming a discontinuity in treatment. Of those patients who did not receive a Pap smear on the first visit and who returned for a second visit, 87 percent saw the same resident. For third visits, 81 percent saw the same doctor. Furthermore, this pattern must be considered in relation to the finding that there was a higher percentage of lower socioeconomic status women (a high-risk group for cervical cancer) with each visit.

Similarly, one might expect that if these doctors were being educated toward a commitment to prevention, third year residents would perform more Pap smears than doctors in earlier stages of training. However, this was not the case. First year residents performed Pap smears on 28.6 percent of their first visit patients but since they had the least access to patients, these doctors accounted for only 5.5 percent of the 253 visits. The bulk of the first visits was divided among the second (43.5 percent) and third (51 percent) year residents. Forty percent of the visits involving second year residents included a Pap smear compared to 22.5 percent for the third year residents. In this program, the second and third years of residency involved more extensive clinical practice than did the first year. Since the duties of second and third year residents were the same, we cannot explain the difference in Pap smear performance except to suggest that the third year residents were not as likely to be "practicing" the procedure.

As described earlier, this training program was organized to model the actual practice of Family Medicine. The residents examined, diagnosed, and prescribed treatment for clinic patients. If they had questions or needed assistance, they consulted the attending staff physicians. While the staff doctors reviewed patient charts to monitor resident performance, the residents primarily practiced on their own initiative. The staff doctors seldom had direct contact with patients coming to the clinic. The only notation about Pap smears regularly entered into patient files were the lab results which were appended to the records. Other comments (e.g., a Pap smear was needed but had not been performed or a Pap smear was not needed because the patient had the procedure performed in another medical setting) were *not* routinely entered into the files. When the charts were reviewed by staff physicians, the absence of information about a patient's Pap history was *not* interpreted as unusual or in need of remedy. This was an unexpected pattern to find in an educational setting oriented toward preventive medicine.

The findings presented to this point suggest that Pap smears were performed most often in this clinic setting when they were requested, required, or convenient. As shown in Table 1, medical reason for the visit was the strongest variable for distinguishing the Pap/no Pap outcome. Of the three reasons for visit, pelvic indicator included conditions which most obviously necessitated or suggested a Pap smear. For example, some patients requested the procedure and therefore made the outcome decision themselves. A Pap smear was required as part of the medical protocol for pregnancy. Also, women who requested a birth control method were likely to receive a Pap smear, especially when birth control pills were prescribed. Pap smears were common with pelvic complaints probably because the procedure either was necessary for a diagnosis (e.g., for irregular vaginal bleeding) or was convenient (i.e., the patient was undressed and/or the doctor was examining the pelvic region) (Fisher, 1984). The second reason for visit, general physical, involved a more thorough examination of the patient (i.e., across body systems) to establish health or to diagnose or treat illness. The Pap smear procedure was less frequently a part of this examining process. In contrast, nonpelvic complaint visits seldom included Pap smears. These were specific medical problems (e.g., sore throat, ear ache) which normally did not require a pelvic examination or a more detailed physical exam for diagnosis or treatment. There was probably an element of convenience involved in these decisions. General physical patients were usually undressed, while nonpelvic complaint patients were generally not undressed, especially below the waist (Fisher, 1984).

Targeting High-Risk Patients

If preventive screening programs are to be cost-effective, high-risk groups must be targeted for tests. Of course, in this case, one might argue that because Appalachia has the highest cervical cancer rate in the country, Pap smears should be a routine feature of medical exams and/or visits. However, this is the ideal, not the reality. While this clinical setting may not have been as conducive to the performance of Pap smears as first expected, there is some suggestion that women with certain high-risk characteristics did receive Pap smears more frequently. Although we have no evidence concerning several known risk factors (e.g., age at first coitus) and only indirect evidence about others (e.g., socioeconomic status), we can make a few general statements about targeting in this case.

The profile of the Pap patient group was described in the results section. Certain of the profiled traits may correspond to known cervical cancer risk factors. For example, previous studies (Handy & Weiben, 1965; Marshall, 1965; Walton et al., 1979) pointed to lower socioeconomic status women (having no insurance and being in the 9–12 education category in our study), Black women (non-white in our study), and women in the 40–50 age group as being at high risk. Other studies (Canadian Task Force, 1976, 1982; Draper, 1982) have shown that younger, sexually active women are also at risk (patients under 20 and students in our study). However, as we noted earlier, some of the profiled relationships were relatively weak.

The only consistent indication in our data that high-risk women were targeted were the age categories most often screened. As shown in Table 1, the odds ratios for receiving a Pap smear were highest in the under 20 and 40–49 age groups. Obviously, the 40–49 age category is a high-risk group displaying many gynecological problems (Marshall, 1965). Furthermore, the assumption that our under 20 age group received more Pap smears because it was at greater risk seems to be supported when other risk factors are examined (e.g., students, singles, Blacks, low education and income). However, the Canadian Task Force studies (1976, 1982) also stated that women born from 1955 on belong to high-risk birth cohorts (i.e., assumes early onset of sexual activity and multiple partners) and that annual screening was justifiable until age 35. Therefore, it may be that only a portion of the "young" high-risk group in our study received Pap smears.

While the age variable does offer some evidence for targeting, we must reiterate that the medical reason for the visit was by far the strongest determinant of the Pap/no Pap outcome. Women whose reason for visit was a pelvic indicator had the highest odds of receiving a Pap smear. This was the case in each age category. This leads us to suggest that the findings in this case most strongly support the claim that Pap smears were performed when they were requested, required, or convenient. At the very least, we would expect that more Pap smears would be performed in such a structured, educational setting.

As mentioned in the introduction, the medical care system in this country continues to be criticized for a lack of orientation toward prevention. Concern is focused on the possible health consequences for the population. With our study, we offer some evidence for this critical point of view. However, while the findings are interesting, this was essentially an exploratory study. A more comprehensive analysis of preventive procedures requires a consideration of factors other than those studied here. Further research needs to consider additional patient variables (especially sociodemographic measures), resident training modes, medical specialties, practice settings, and sociodemographic and attitudinal variables for examining physicians.

FOOTNOTES

1. A Pap smear is a sampling of cells from the cervix. The procedure can provide information on abnormal cell changes which may be precursors of cervical cancer. Even older women who have had hysterectomies need to have Pap smears since these abnormal cell changes can also occur in vaginal tissue. Furthermore, a Pap smear is normally accompanied by a pelvic examination which can discover other life-threatening conditions (e.g., ovarian cysts).

2. Approximately 465,000 new cases of invasive cancer are expected to occur in 1985 in the United States, including 15,000 cases of cervical cancer and 36,000 cases of endometrium cancer (cancer of the lining of the womb). For patients diagnosed early, the survival rate for cervical cancer is 80–90 percent. In fact, for patients diagnosed before the disease has become invasive (cancer-in-situ), the survival rate is virtually 100 percent. However, without early detection, the five year survival rate for cervical cancer patients, white and Black, is 62 percent (American Cancer Society, 1986).

3. By August 31, 1982, the family practice program described in this study had produced 46 graduates. Forty of the doctors are currently practicing in the state. Three are elsewhere in the rural Southeast, while 3 are in rural areas outside the region.

4. The federal government's definition of a "medically underserved area" is based upon several criteria, including number of non-Federal physicians/100,000 population, number of primary care physicians/100,000 population, number of specialists/100,000 population, and number of hospital beds/1000 population.

5. In this paper, we use the terms "doctor" and "resident" interchangeably to refer to the family practice residents. There were 22 family practice residents in the program during the data collection stage of this study. Five were first year residents, 7 were second year, and 10 were in their third year of residency. Twenty doctors were male and all were white. Unless a specific doctor was requested, new patients were allocated by rotation to available residents.

6. U.S. Department of Health, Education, and Welfare statistics establish the Pap smear as a well-used procedure. In a 1975 study, approximately 50 percent of the women over the age of 17 reported having had the procedure during the previous year.

REFERENCES

American Cancer Society. (1986). *Cancer facts and figures*. New York: American Cancer Society.

Boyes, D.A. (1972). Guest editorial. *Mayo Clinic Proceedings*, *47*, 533.

Boyes, D.A., Nichols, T.M., Miller, A.M., & Worth, A.J. (1977). Recent results from the

British Columbia screening program for cervical cancer. *American Journal of Obstetrics and Gynecology*. *128*, 692–693.

Brown, A.J. (1976). Awareness and use of cervical cancer tests in a southern Appalachian community. *Public Health Reports*, *91*, 236–242.

Burns, E.L., Hammond, E., Percy, C., Seidman, H., & Gorski, T. (1968). Detection of uterine cancer: Results of a community program of 17 years. *Cancer*, *22*, 1108–1119.

Canadian Task Force Appointed by the Conference of Deputy Ministers of Health. (1976). Cervical Cancer screening programs. The Walton report. *Canadian Medical Association Journal*, *114*, 1003–1033.

Canadian Task Force Appointed by the Conference of Deputy Ministers of Health. (1982). Cervical cancer screening programs: Summary of the 1982 Canadian Task Force Report. *Canadian Medical Association Journal*, *127*, 581–589.

Christopherson, W.M., Parker, J., Mendez, W., & Lundin, F. (1970). Cervix cancer control in Louisville, Kentucky. *Cancer*, *26*, 29–38.

Cramer, D.W. (1974). The role of cervical cytology in the declining morbidity and mortality of cervical cancer. *Cancer*, *34*, 2018–2027.

Dickinson, L., Mussey, M., & Kurland, L. (1972). Evaluation of the effectiveness of cytologic screening for cervical cancer. *Mayo Clinic Proceedings*, *47*, 534–544.

Draper, G.J., & Cook, G.A. (1983). Changing patterns of cervical cancer rates. *British Medical Journal*, *287*, 510–512.

Draper, G.J. (1982). Screening for cervical cancer: Revised policy. The recommendations of the DHSS Committee on Gynaecological Cytology. *British Journal of Family Planning*, *8*, 95–100.

Emerson, J. (1970). Behavior in private places: Sustaining definitions of reality in gynecological examinations. In H.P. Dreitzel (Editor), *Recent sociology no. 2*. London: Macmillian, pp. 73–113.

Fleiss, J.L. (1981). *Statistical methods for rates and proportions: Second edition*. New York: John Wiley & Sons.

Fisher, S. (1986). *In the Patient's Best Interest: Women and the Politics of Medical Decision*. New Brunswick, NJ: Rutgers University Press.

Flannery, M.A. (1982). Primary care in rural Appalachia: Simple living and hard choices. *The Hastings Center Report*, (August), 9–12.

Fowinkle, E. (1975). *Health in Tennessee: A statistical overview: Second edition*. Nashville: Tennessee Office of Comprehensive Health Planning.

Fruchter, R.G., Boyce, J., & Hunt, M. (1980). Missed opportunities for early diagnosis of cancer of the cervix. *American Journal of Public Health*, *70*, 418–420.

Graham, S., & Schotz, W. (1979). Epidemiology of cancer of the cervix in Buffalo, New York. *Journal of the National Cancer Institute*, *63*, (1), 23–27.

Handy, V.H., & Wieben, E. (1965). Detection of cancer of the cervix: A public health approach. *Obstetrics and Gynecology*, *25*, 348–355.

Kegeles, S.S. (1967). Attitudes and behavior of the public regarding cervical cytology: Current findings and new directions for research. *Journal of Chronic Disease*, *20*, 911–922.

Kleinman, J.C. (1979). Death rates from cervical cancer by health service area, 1968–1979. *Statistical Notes for Health Planning* (Department of Health, Education, and Welfare). Washington, DC: Government Printing Office, (August).

Knopf, A. (1976). Changes in women's opinions about cancer. *Social Science and Medicine*, *10*, 191–195.

Knowles, J.H. (1977). Doing better and feeling worse: Health in the United States. *Daedalus*, (Winter), 1–7, 57–80.

Lundin, F.E., Christopherson, W., Mendez, W., & Parker, J. (1965). Morbidity from cervical cancer: Effects of cervical cytology and socioeconomic status. *Journal of the National Cancer Institute*, *35*, 1015–1025.

Lynge, E. (1983). Regional trends in incidence of cervical cancer in Denmark in relation to local smear-taking activity. *International Journal of Epidemiology*, *12*, 405–413.
Magee, J. (1975). The pelvic examination: A view from the other end of the table. *Annals of Internal Medicine*, *83*, 563–564.
Marshall, C.E. (1965). Effect of cytologic screening on the incidence of invasive carcinoma of the cervix in a semi-closed community. *Cancer*, *18*, 153–156.
Marx, J.L. (1979). The annual Pap smear: An idea whose time has come? *Science*, *205*(13), 177–178.
Mason, T.J., & McKay, F.W. (1969). *U.S. cancer mortality by county 1950–1969* (Department of Health, Education, and Welfare). Washington, DC: Government Printing Office.
McCurtis, J.W. (1979). Social contact factors in the diffusion of cervical cytology among Mexican-Americans in Los Angeles County, California. *Social Science and Medicine*, *13*, 807–811.
Ob, Gyn News. (1983). Routine Pap advised regardless of patient's presenting complaints. *17*(20), 51.
Sall, S., Pineda, A., Sedlis, A., & Stone, M. (1968). Impact of a cytologic screening program on a gynecologic malignancy service. *Cancer*, *22*, 1120–1125.
Shulman, J., Leyton, M., & Hamilton, R. (1974). The Papanicolaou smear: An insensitive case-finding procedure. *American Journal of Obstetrics and Gynecology*, *120*, 446–451.
Sidel, V.W., & Sidel, R. (1981). Health care and medical care in the United States. In P. Conrad and R. Kern (Editors). *The Sociology of Health and Illness*. New York: St. Martin's Press, pp. 203–219.
Taylor, R. (1982). The politics of prevention. *Social Policy*, *13*(1), 32–41.
Terris, M. (1980). Prevention services and medical care: The costs and benefits of basic change. *Bulletin New York Academy of Medicine*, *56*(1), 180–189.
Timonen, S., Nieminen, U., & Kauraniemi, T. (1974). Cervical screening. *The Lancet*, *1* (March), 401–402.
U.S. Department of Health, Education, and Welfare, Public Health Service, National Center for Health Statistics. (1975). Characteristics of females ever having a Pap smear and interval since last Pap smear, United States, 1973. *Monthly Vital Statistics Report*, *24*(7), 76–1120. Washington, DC: Government Printing Office.
Veal, K.F. (1983). University hospital fund gives hope to women with cancer. *Knoxville News-Sentinel*, April 24, 1C.
Walton, L.A., Kernodle, W., & Hulka, B. (1979). Factors influencing the occurence of advanced cervical carcinoma. *Southern Medical Journal*, *72*, 808–811.

The Impact of Mastectomy on Self-Concept and Social Function: A Combined Cross-Sectional and Longitudinal Study With Comparison Groups

Doris T. Penman, PhD
Joan R. Bloom, PhD
Sophia Fotopoulos, PhD
Mary R. Cook, PhD
Jimmie C. Holland, MD
Christopher Gates, MD
Daphne Flamer, PhD
Benjamin Murawski, PhD
Robert Ross
Ursula Brandt, PhD
Larry R. Muenz, ScD
David Pee, M. Phil

Doris T. Penman is Deputy Director for Clinical Services, Ulster County Mental Health Services, 276 Fair St., Box 1800, Kingston, NY 12401. Joan R. Bloom is Professor, School of Public Health, University of California, 409 Warren Hall, Berkeley, CA 94970. Sophia Fotopoulos is Director, Research Grants and Contracts, American University, 4400 Massachusettes Ave., NW, Washington, D.C. 20016. Mary R. Cook is Head, Biobehavioral Sciences Section, Midwest Research Institute, Kansas City, MO 64110. Jimmie C. Holland is Professor of Psychiatry, Cornell University Medical College and Chief, Psychiatry Service, Memorial Sloan-Kettering Cancer Center, 1275 York Ave., New York, NY 10021. Christopher Gates, 34 Hawthorne Rd., Brookline, MA 02146, is Consulting Psychiatrist, Brigham and Women's Hospital, Boston, MA. Daphne Flamer is Manager, Shaklee Corporation, 444 Market St., San Francisco, CA 94111. Benjamin Murawski is Associate Professor of Psychology, Department of Psychiatry, Harvard Medical School, Brigham and Women's Hospital, 75 Francis St., Boston, MA 02115. Robert Ross, 240 Selby Lane, Atherton, CA 94025, is with American Healthway Systems, Menlo Park, CA. Ursula Brandt is Assistant Professor of Psychology, Department of Psychiatry, Harvard Medical School, Brigham and Women's Hospital, 75 Francis St., Boston, MA 02115. Larry R. Muenz is Senior Statistician, SRA Technology, Inc., 4700 King St., Alexandria, VA 22302. David Pee is Biostatistician, Information Management Services, Inc., 1400 Spring St., Suite 500, Silver Spring, MD 20910. Address reprint request to Joan R. Bloom at the School of Public Health, 409 Warren Hall, University of California, Berkely, CA 94970.

This study was supported by the National Cancer Institute under contracts N01-CN-65311, 55312, 55313, 55314, and 55214 to the Psychological Aspects of Breast Cancer

ABSTRACT. Self-concept and social function following radical, modified radical or simple mastectomy for Stage I or II breast cancer, breast biopsy for benign breast disease, cholecystectomy or no operative procedure were measured across a fifteen-month period in a cross-sectional design and across a twelve-month period in a repeated measures design. Women selected for study were without other pre-existing mental or physical illness. The degree of disability observed following mastectomy was considerably less than previously reported in uncontrolled studies, with the incidence of actual disturbance extremely small. Women receiving adjuvant therapies following mastectomy, but not women treated by mastectomy alone, reported significantly more body-image dissatisfaction and feminine self-image concerns than the comparison groups. The findings refute previously published impressions of severe psychosocial maladjustments following mastectomy. The study suggests that post-mastectomy women vulnerable to poorer outcome would be those with lower expectations of good quality social support, other present life stressors, other pre-existing chronic diseases, and a disposition to believe in life outcomes as less under their own control.

Breast cancer, the most common cancer in women, is a serious disease that continues to take its toll despite intensive research and aggressive treatment. Mastectomy is the oldest and most common treatment for early breast cancer and even with the advent of newer breast-sparing procedures will continue to be a major treatment modality. Radiotherapy or chemotherapy as adjuvant therapies following surgery have produced additional gains in survival for women with Stage II disease. As efforts at early cancer detection and aggressive treatment intensify, the impact of mastectomy and adjuvant treatment on women's psychosocial health is therefore a subject of serious and continuing concern.

The literature on psychosocial aspects of mastectomy is sizeable and has been summarized in a number of annotated bibliographies and literature reviews (Lewis and Bloom, 1978–79; Myerowitz, 1980; National Cancer Institute, 1978; Taylor and Levin, 1976a). Conveyed in much of this literature is the message that the combined impact of cancer and mastectomy produces, in a significant number

---

(PABC) Study Group at the following research sites: Midwest Research Institute, Kansas City, MO; Montefiore Hospital and Medical Center, Bronx, NY; Peter Bent Brigham Hospital, Boston, MA; Stadford Research Institute International, Menlo Park, CA and West Coast Cancer Foundation, San Franciso, CA. The authors recognize the following National Cancer Institute staff for their support: Joseph Cullen, PhD, Lawrence Burke, MSW, Wendy Schain, EdD, Shepard Insel, EdD, Sandra Levy, PhD, Lillian Gigliotti, PhD and Larry Kessler, ScD.

of women, a measurable psychosocial morbidity. These women are then potentially at risk for, among other things, an impaired body image, diminished femininity, self-depreciation, family disequilibrium, marital and social withdrawal and workplace rejection.

The actual assessment of psychosocial morbidity is a difficult task, as is any research endeavor involving a complex set of psychophysiological relationships. Impact of the cancer surgery must be distinguished from the impact of surgery itself. The surgical loss of a breast with its implications for the feminine psyche and body image must be distinguished from the impact of surgery for a threatening breast condition which did not result in breast loss. Sociodemographic and other pre-existing life factors relevant to impact must be considered in measurement and care must be taken to avoid confounding the effect of mastectomy with serious pre-existing mental or physical illness. Evaluation must also consider the stages of the recovery process itself and the age of the patient.

Studies to date have lacked the necessary controls because of the difficulty of mounting a research effort with a sufficiently large study group to permit measurement and control of the number of relevant variables.

In 1977, the National Cancer Institute, Division of Cancer Control and Prevention, initiated and funded a large, comprehensive, multi-center prospective study to evaluate psychological, psychosocial and physical consequences of mastectomy in women with breast cancer. Five institutions collaborated: The Midwest Research Institute (Kansas City, MO), the Stanford Research Institute (Menlo Park, CA), the West Coast Cancer Foundation (San Francisco, CA), the Montefiore Hospital and Medical Center (Bronx, NY) and the Peter Bent Brigham Hospital (Boston, MA). The broad-based comparison research approach that the NCI support made possible permitted a more definitive assessment of the phychosocial and physical morbidity associated with breast cancer surgery than had ever previously been undertaken. The study design provided for equal numbers of women with Stage I or II breast cancer so that these groups could be evaluated separately. Additionally, the study design permitted comparison with women who had just undergone cholecystectomy and breast biopsy, as well as with women who had not recently had surgery at all. In addition to its goal of defining psychosocial morbidity more precisely, the study aimed to identify predictors of psychosocial morbidity within the breast cancer group and to develop a morbidity-risk index.

A combined cross-sectional and longitudinal (repeated measures) design was selected which when implemented provided data on 1,715 women gathered at 61 hospitals in 11 states on a large set of predictor and outcome variables related to psychological, social and physical function. This paper presents the self-concept and social function outcomes of the study, providing the most comprehensive and best-controlled study of such outcomes to date.

METHODS

Study Design

A combined cross-sectional and longitudinal study design was chosen to overcome the inherent weaknesses of either design alone. Cross-sectional designs produce uncontrollable sources of variance because a different sample is used at each time point, and longitudinal designs, while usually more powerful, are subject to the confounding effects of repeated testings of the same sample. When both designs are employed, each can serve as a control for the other. If the same patterns of response are observed in both designs, confidence in the results is increased; if different patterns are found, the differences can lead to identification of error.

The use of comparison groups in the designs was deemed essential because it is known that surgery itself has profound psychological effects, even when the underlying disorder poses little threat to life.

The study sample was collected as a stratified sample, with each collaborating institution contributing pre-determined numbers of participants by age decade per study group. Each institution's assignment was made so that equal numbers by decade were assessed within specified time intervals since surgery. The cross sectional component of the study used a different sample at each of five post-surgical time intervals. The groups which served as the sample for the first post-surgical time interval in the cross-sectional study also served as the longitudinal sample, which was followed across three additional time intervals over the year. The control for age was important because most available assessment instruments are standardized without norms for age and the known tendency for differential responses by age must be taken into account. Therefore, all groups included women in four decades: 30–39, 40–49, 50–59 and 60–69. While breast cancer is a disease of older, rather than younger women, the choice of these four decades was prompted by concern over ability to locate sufficient subjects in all surgical groups by age, and an unequal distribution of elderly populations in the communities where the studies were undertaken. The number collected at each age group was predetermined by hospital census data per collaborating institution. Both designs employed time-since-surgery as time blocks: up to 3, 6, 9 or 12 months since surgery in the longitudinal component with an additional interval of up to 15 months in the cross-sectional. The study design is summarized in Table 1.

The outcome variables reported in this paper and their measures

Table 1

Study Design and Accruals

	Time Block Months				
	0-3	3-6	6-9	9-12	12-15
Cross-sectional component (N=1,715)					
Study group					
Mastectomy + adjuv	28	45	42	43	50
Mastectomy only	117	82	90	83	81
Cholecystectomy	90	59	64	61	76
Benign breast biopsy	87	68	65	71	74
No surgery	90	123	38	41	47
Longitudinal component (N=412)*					
Study group					
Mastectomy + adjuv	28	28	20	25	
Mastectomy only	117	99	98	101	
Cholecystectomy	90	79	72	79	
Benign breast biopsy	87	77	73	73	
No surgery	90	86	84	84	

*The women followed across time in the longitudinal component are the same women who appear in the 0-3 months time block of the cross-sectional component.

are summarized in Table 2. The study design and comparisons were formulated to test the hypothesis that on each selected single indicator of self-concept and social function, the mastectomy groups

Table 2

Summary of Measures Used to Assess Psychosocial Outcomes

Outcome Variables	Measures	Number of Items
Self-esteem impairment	Self-esteem Scale (Rosenberg, 1965)	10
Body image dissatisfaction	Body Image Scale (Berscheid, 1972)	22
Feminine self-image concerns	Feminine Self-Image Scale from: Personal Problem Checklist (Schain, 1977)	4
Intimacy concerns	Intimacy Scale from: Personal Problem Checklist (Schain, 1977)	3
Social health	Social Health Index from: National Health Survey (Ware, 1976)	9
Dysfunctional interaction with family	Interaction with Family Members Scale from: Sickness Impact Profile (Gilson, et al., 1975)	10
Personal & social life events stress	Personal and Social Changes Scale from: Social Readjustment Rating Scale (Holmes and Rahe, 1967)	18
Workplace life events stress	Work Changes Scale from: Social Re-adjustment Rating Scale (Holmes and Rahe, 1976)	15
Social role functions impairment	Role Impairment Scales from: Psychiatric Evaluation Form (Spitzer, et al., 1968)	5
Daily life activities impairment	Social Isolation and Daily Routine-Leisure Time Impairment Scales from: Psychiatric Evaluation Form (Spitzer, et al., 1968)	2

Note. All but the last two variables were assessed by self-report measures administered in booklet form. Impairment in social role functions and daily life activities were clinician-rated following a structured interview.

would show a measureable and significant difference in the direction of poorer outcome from the no-surgery, or referent, group which would be greater than that of the non-mastectomy surgical comparison groups.

A set of predictor variables was chosen to control for individual differences in demographic, psychological or social characteristics that might differentially affect outcome. These are summarized in Table 3.

Subjects

Sequential cases of women who had undergone simple, modified radical or radical mastectomy, cholecystectomy or breast biopsy were screened according to the criteria shown in Table 4. To prevent the confounding of findings by pre-existing illnesses, the exclusion criteria eliminated from study individuals with obvious mental or debilitating physical illness.

All selection procedures were the same for each institution. Women appropriate for study who gave verbal permission were put in touch with research staff by screening personnel. The rate of refusal was very small and we do not consider it contributed a substantial bias. Subjects were accumulated until the equivalent required numbers for all study cells at each contributing institution were filled. Subjects for the no-surgery comparison group were recruited through study subjects or from local neighborhoods to approximate the socio-demographic characteristics of the other study groups. Subjects were paid for expenses incurred.

Selected characteristics of the study sample are displayed in Table 5. Of the total mastectomy group, 31 percent received adjuvant chemotherapy, radiotherapy, or both, following mastectomy and 69 percent received no adjuvant treatment. For data analyses, mastectomy subjects were divided into two groups; those receiving adjuvant therapy and those not receiving adjuvant therapy.

Study data were gathered between January, 1978 and July, 1979. Longitudinal subjects were assessed four times, cross-sectional subjects once. Assessments were smoothly distributed across time intervals. Time of recruitment was the starting point for the no-surgery group. Before any first assessment, the study rationale and procedures were explained to subjects in detail and written consent was obtained. Findings presented in this paper were obtained by two assessment techniques: a self-report assessment in

Table 3

Summary of Measures Used as Predictor Variables or Covariates in the Analysis of Psychosocial Outcomes

Independent Variables	Measures	Number of Items
Social status	Four Factor Index of Social Status (Hollingshead)	4
Chronic medical conditions	Chronic Conditions Inventory from: National Health Survey (Ware, 1976)	23
Social contacts	Social Contacts Index from: National Health Survey (Ware, 1976)	3
Group participation	Group Participation Index from: National Health Survey (Ware, 1976)	2
Lack of social supports	Perceived Social Support Scale (Flamer, 1977)	15
Life events stress	Social Readjustment Rating Scale (Holmes and Rahe, 1967)	75
Locus of control	Locus of Control Scale (Levenson, 1974)	24
Married	Married vs. never married, widowed or divorced	
Employed	Employed vs. unemployed less than one year vs. unemployed for more than one year	
Early loss of parent(s)	One or both parents not present in home until age twelve vs. both parents present	
Overweight	Self-report of overweight as a health condition	

Note. All variables listed were assessed by self-report measures administered in booklet form.

TABLE 4

Study Exclusion Criteria
All Groups
Previous mastectomy
Age < 30, > 69
Inability to read, write or speak English
Incapable of self-care without assistance
History of serious mental illness or use of major psychoactive drugs
History of traditional psychotherapy for three months or more
Any major surgery two years prior to or subsequent to target surgery
History of any type of cancer
Other surgery at time of target surgery
Mastectomy Groups
Extended radical mastectomy or bilateral mastectomy
Tumor other than Stage I or II breast cancer
Previous breast biopsy or mirror biopsy after release from hospital
Evidence of metastasis during study
History of hormonal therapy
Biopsy Group
Bilateral, needle or previous biopsy in last two years
Biopsy positive for cancer
Cholecystectomy Group
Breast biopsy in last two years
No-Surgery Group
Breast biopsy in last two years
Cholecystectomy in last five years

booklet form for all subjects and additional clinician ratings based on structured interview for longitudinal subjects at the first and fourth intervals. Assessments and interviews were conducted at a research site or in the subject's home by female technicians and clinical interviewers. Initial and ongoing training to criterion was provided for interviewer ratings.

TABLE 5

Demographic and Social Data for All Subjects (N = 1,715)

	Percentage Of Subjects		Percentage
Age decade		Living Situation	
30-39	16	with spouse/partner	30
40-49	26	with spouse, children	40
50-59	33	with children, others	15
60-69	25	alone	15
Race		Vocational Status	
White	86	Full or part-time work	54
Black	7	Volunteer work	8
Other	7	Not employed	38
Marital status		Income	
Married	70	5,000 - 14,999	28
Widowed	10	15,000 - 29,999	35
Divorced/separated	12	30,000	18
Never married	8	Unknown	19

Mean years of schooling = 13.4

Outcome Measures

The Self-Esteem Scale (Rosenberg, 1965) consists of 10 items which measure attitudes toward the self such as self-worth, self-criticism and self-acceptance along a favorable to unfavorable continuum. The Body Image Scale (Bersheid, Walster and Bohrnstedt, 1972) as edited by Polivy (1977) consists of 20 body parts and two body qualities which are rated for appearance along a satisfied to dissatisfied continuum. The Feminine Self-Image and Intimacy Scales were identified by a principal components analysis of the Personal Problem Checklist developed by Schain (1977) which addresses concerns particularly voiced by post-mastectomy women but worded without specific reference to breast cancer. The scale differentiated women who had breast reconstruction after surgery from those who did not. The Feminine Self-Image items assess body self-consciousness, sexual attractiveness, feelings of femininity and clothing fit. The Intimacy items address concerns around physical affection, sexual relations and avoidance of close relationships.

The Social Health Index, a composite measure of social ties and activities with family, friends and groups over the past one month is from a set of health indices developed and tested by Ware (1976) for medical care policy research, now published separately (Donald and Ware, 1982). The Interaction with Family Members Scale was extracted from the Sickness Impact Profile, a set of health care outcome measures developed by Gilson, Gilson and Bergner, et al. (1975). Ten scale items in a true-false format describe behavioral expressions of physical illness as it affects daily behavior in relation to family members. The Personal-Social and Workplace Changes Scales were extracted from the Social Readjustment Rating Scale (Holmes and Rahe, 1967) which quantifies the stress impact of a set of common life changes by weighting items for the degree of readjustment required. The 18 items of the Personal-Social Scale cover changes in personal habits, activities, beliefs and relationships as well as personal achievements and losses. The Workplace Changes Scale includes 15 items covering changes in work type, hours, conditions and responsibilities as well as work problems and work loss. The time frame used for these items was the past three months.

The Role Impairment, Social Isolation and Daily Routine-Leisure Time Scales of the Psychiatric Evaluation Form (Spitzer, Endicott, Mesnikoff and Cohen, 1978) are rated following a structured interview designed to elicit functional ability and comfort in carrying out the social roles in which the subject is engaged and in routine or leisure-time tasks, activities and involvements.

Predictor Measures

The Four Factor Index of Social Status (Hollingshead), supplied to us by the author in 1977, combines the education and occupation of an individual and spouse to provide a measure of the individual's social status, taking into account retirement, divorce and widowhood. The Chronic Conditions Inventory is a 23-item list of chronic medical conditions such as arthritis, asthma, diabetes, sinus trouble and varicose veins. The index controls for symptom variance unrelated to the target surgery. Social Contacts and Group Participation Scales are sub-scales of the Social Health Index. Both indices were developed for use in health policy research (Ware, 1976; Donald and Ware, 1982). The Perceived Social Support Scale (Flamer, 1977) is a list of 15 basic emotional and social supports individuals identify as available or unavailable from people close to them. Such social supports are considered to moderate the effects of stress. The Social Readjustment Rating Scale (Holmes and Rahe, 1967) described earlier was used to account for possible sources of distress other than the target surgeries during any preceding three months. Weights for the most-recently added of the 55 items were received by personal communication from Rahe. For use in some analyses, a shorter (adjusted) scale was used to avoid duplication of content in independent and dependent measures. The Locus of Control Scales developed by Levenson (1974) measure the extent to which people feel that the events of their lives are under their personal control or are controlled by others or chance. The concept was included as a variable because such expectancy beliefs are thought to mediate an individual's response to stressful experiences. Levenson's eight-item scales isolate three control dimensions: Internal, Powerful Others and Chance. For economy, the scales were combined for longitudinal analyses.

The sociodemographic characteristics of being married and employed were also included as predictors in the analyses of both study components. In the cross-sectional data analyses, social groups participation and social ties were included as predictors as was early loss of one or both parents, included to test the assumption that an early loss experience might render an individual more vulnerable to loss of a body part. Overweight was used as a predictor of poorer outcome in both analysis models for the body image dissatisfaction outcome only.

The hypotheses to be examined using the predictor variables were that lower social status, greater number of chronic medical conditions, fewer social supports, greater life events stress, less internal locus of control expectancy, fewer group memberships and social contact activities, unemployed status and early parental loss would all contribute to poorer psychosocial outcomes.

Statistical Methods

All scales used in the study were scored as determined by their originators. For uniformity of final data presentation, some scales were reversed so as to have the numerically higher scores represent greater distress or dysfunction, as indicated by the variable names, except for social health which was scored according to original determination.

For the analysis of the cross-sectional data, a multiple regression model was employed, with hierarchical inclusion of the three sets of stratification variables: study group, age by decade and time since surgery in time block form. The no-surgery group, the 30–39 age decade and the last time block, incorporated into the model via dummy or indicator variable coding schemes, served as the referent groups. Standard guidelines were employed for determining stepwise inclusion of the predictor variables.

A Repeated Measures Analysis of Variance with covariates utilizing the UCLA BMDP Program was used to test the study hypotheses using the longitudinal data. Because the repeated measures analysis model required valid data at all four time points and has fewer degrees of freedom, only the most strategic covariates were chosen in order to prevent unncessary loss of subjects due to missing data.

Of the 412 women who participated in the longitudinal study, 88% were assessed at all four time blocks. Longitudinal subjects tested three or fewer times were excluded from evaluation of the self-report data, but were included in the analysis of clinical interview data if they were present for those assessments.

The mastectomy group was divided between those women who received adjuvant therapy (chemotherapy, radiotherapy or both) and those who did not.

Findings significant at $p < .05$ (two-tailed) are reported, constituting conservative probability estimates because of the a priori predictions of the directions of all findings except for the stratification variables of age and time, and for marital status among the predictors.

Tables 6 and 8 show the effect on psychosocial outcome of surgical group membership (in relation to the no surgery group), time since surgery (in relation to the time interval furthest from surgery) and age decade (in relation to the youngest decade) after controlling for significant predictor variables in the cross-sectional component of the study. Tables 7 and 9 show results of the longitudinal component of the study, indicating study group and time effects on outcome after adjustments have been made for age and predictor variables. Figures 1–3 display the group means over time for study outcomes after these adjustments have been made in the longitudinal component of the study.

RESULTS

Self-Esteem Impairment

Neither of the mastectomy groups (Mastectomy + Adjuvant and Mastectomy Only) reported significantly lower self-esteem in the year post-surgery than the referent group (No-Surgery) or the comparison surgical groups (Cholecystectomy and Biopsy). As averaged across time blocks, no significant group differences were found in either the cross-sectional or longitudinal component of the study (Tables 6 and 7). However, as shown in Figure 1, the overall decrease in self-esteem over time of the Mastectomy + Adjuvant group, which showed poorer self-esteem at the end of the year than it did in the initial assessment raises the possibility of significant sequelae emerging after a longer period of time. We did find that women in their forties, fifties and sixties reported significantly higher self-esteem than the referent age group (women 30–39). No effect due to time alone was observed.

Significant predictors of lower self-esteem for women across all groups in both study components were perceived lack of social support, the magnitude of life change stress during a preceding three-month period and locus of control. The more that women viewed their life outcomes as less under their own personal control and more contingent on others more powerfully placed than themselves, the lower their self-esteem. The variables in the regression equation explained 13 percent of the variation in self-esteem.

Body Image Dissatisfaction

The Mastectomy + Adjuvant group reported significantly more dissatisfaction with their body image than the No-Surgery referent group (Tables 6 and 7, Figure 1). This finding was significant in the cross-sectional component of the study but not in the longitudinal component, due to larger estimated standard errors. The magnitude of this difference, however, was small and explained only about one percent of the total variation in self-esteem. Mastectomy alone did not create a significant negative impact on overall body satisfaction in relation to the No-Surgery, Cholecystectomy and Biopsy groups. No effect due to age was found on this measure. There was a time effect in the cross-sectional component; dissatisfaction with body image across groups was greatest in the first post-surgical time block.

Table 6

Multiple Regressions of Self-concept Outcomes on Group, Time, Age and Predictor Variables (Cross-sectional Component)

Variable in Regression	Self-esteem Impairment	Body Image Dissatisfaction	Feminine Self-image Concerns	Intimacy Concerns
Group				
Mastectomy + adj	NS	.09**	.13***	NS
Mastectomy only	NS	NS	NS	NS
Cholecystectomy	NS	NS	NS	NS
Biopsy	NS	NS	-.10***	NS
Time block	NS	.07*	-.08**	NS
Age 40 - 49	-.10**	NS	-.08*	NS
50 - 59	-.12***	NS	-.09**	-.06*
60 - 69	-.12***	NS	-.20***	-.17***
Social status	NS	NS	NS	NS
Chronic conditions	NS	.15***	.12***	NS
Social contacts	NS	NS	NS	NS
Group participation	NS	NS	-.05*	NS
Lack of supports	.20***	.18***	.19***	.36***
Life events stress	.15***	NS	.16***	.16***
Locus of control				
Internal	.13***	.10***	NS	NS
Powerful others	.12***	.06**	.12***	.11***
Chance	NS	NS	NS	NS
Married	NS	NS	NS	NS
Employed	NS	NS	NS	NS
Early loss of parent(s)	NS	.07**	.05*	.05*
Overweight	---	.28***	---	---

Note. Numbers are betas. Significance levels for groups are in relation to No-surgery, for time to the 12-15 month block, and for age to the 30-39 decade. For locus of control, higher scores indicate greater control expectancies. Where time block is significant, it is for the 0-3 month time block.

* $p < .05$. ** $p < .01$. *** $p < .001$ NS=not significant

Table 7

Repeated Measures Analysis of Variance for Self-concept Outcomes Showing Main Effects and Direction of Covariate Effects (Longitudinal Component).

Analysis Variables	Self-esteem Impairment	Body Image Dissatisfaction	Feminine Self-image Concerns	Intimacy Concerns
Main Effects				
Group	NS	NS	$p < .001$	NS
Time	NS	NS	NS	NS
Group x Time	NS	NS	NS	NS
Covariates				
Age 40 - 49	-**	NS	NS	NS
50 - 59	-*	NS	NS	NS
60 - 69	-**	NS	-*	NS
Social Status	NS	NS	NS	NS
Chronic conditions	NS	+**	+*	NS
Lack of supports	+***	+***	+***	+***
Life events stress	+**	NS	+*	+***
Locus of control	+***	+*	+***	NS
Married	NS	---	NS	NS
Overweight	---	+***	---	---

Note. Significance levels for age are in relation to age decade 30-39. For locus of control, higher scores indicate greater external control expectancies.

* $p < .05$ ** $p < .01$. *** $p < .001$. NS=not significant

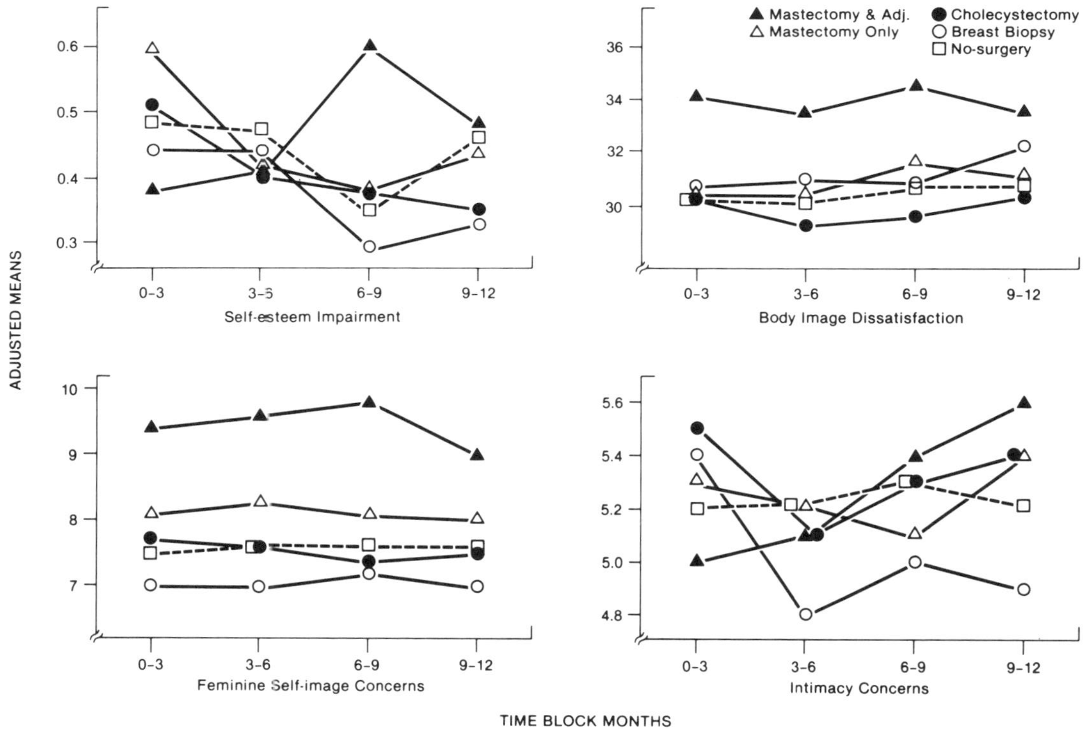

FIGURE 1. Mean scores, covariate adjusted, by time block for self-concept outcomes (longitudinal component).

The most important predictor of body image dissatisfaction in both study components was overweight. Other determinants across groups in both models were the anticipation of fewer social supports being available, a greater number of concurrent chronic medical conditions and locus of control. The more women viewed life outcomes as less under their personal control or determined by more influential others, the poorer their body image. Early loss, a predictor used in the regression equation, was also associated with poorer body image. The variables included in the regression equation explained 19 percent of the variation in body image dissatisfaction.

Feminine Self-Image Concerns

The Mastectomy + Adjuvant group expressed significantly greater self-image concerns related to feeling feminine and sexually attractive than the No-Surgery referent group. The Mastectomy Only group was not distinguishable from the No-Surgery and Cholecystectomy groups. Women in the Biopsy group reported significantly less concern than the referent group. These differences were observed in both study components (Tables 6 and 7) and consistently across time in the repeated measures analysis (Figure 1). Again, the magnitude of these differences was small and accounted for only approximately one percent of the variance in the measure. There was an effect of age; in the cross-sectional component women in the three older decades were significantly less likely to express such concerns than younger women. In the longitudinal component, this finding was observed for the oldest decade only. An effect due to time since surgery was found in the cross-sectional component; feminine self-image concerns were least reported at the first post-surgical assessment.

Predictors significant in both study components were perceived lack of social supports, concurrent chronic medical conditions, the stress of recent life changes and locus of control (as an attribution to more powerful others). Analyzed in the cross-sectional study alone and significant were early parental loss, associated with greater feminine self-image concern, and participation in groups or clubs, associated with less. All variables explained 17 percent of the variance in the regression analysis.

Intimacy Concerns

On this measure of concerns related to physical affection, sexual relations and avoidance of close relationships, there were no differences among study groups (Tables 6 and 7). The Mastectomy + Adjuvant group however, showed a consistent rise in such concerns over time (Figure 1), again suggesting the need for following women longer than one year. No time effect was found. Age was a factor in the regression analysis. Women in their fifties and sixties were less likely to express intimacy concerns than the younger women.

Predictors of intimacy concerns in both study components were having fewer social supports and experiencing greater life events adjustments. In the regression analysis, locus of control (again as an attribution to more powerful others) and early parental loss were associated with greater intimacy concerns. Twenty-one percent of the variance in the regression equation was explained by the study variables.

Social Health

Compared to the No-surgery group, all surgery groups in the cross-sectional component except the Mastectomy + Adjuvant group had poorer social health, as indicated by this measure of social ties and frequency of interaction with relatives, friends and social groups (Table 8). The difference was small and explained less than two percent of the variance in social health scores. These differences did not reach significance in the longitudinal study component (Table 9, Figure 2). No time or age effects were found.

Across groups in both study components, women of higher social status (based on education and occupation) were more likely to report social activity and women with poorer social supports, less activity. In the cross-sectional component of the study, locus of control was a significant predictor; women reported poorer social health when they expected less personal control and more chance events to play a role in their lives. Also, early loss and employment, entered as variables in the cross-sectional regression analysis were negative contributors to social health; employment was perhaps significant because employed women have less time to devote to such activities. The variables in the regression analysis explained 11 percent of the variance in social health.

Table 8
Multiple Regression of Social Function Outcomes on Group, Time, Age and Predictor Variables (Cross-sectional Component).

Variable in Regression	Social Health	Dysfunctional Interaction with Family	Personal and Social Life Events Stress	Workplace Life Events Stress
Group				
Mastectomy + adj	NS	NS	NS	NS
Mastectomy only	-.09**	NS	NS	NS
Cholecstectomy	-.10**	NS	NS	NS
Biopsy	-.10***	NS	NS	NS
Time block	NS	NS	NS	NS
Age 40 - 49	NS	NS	-.22***	NS
50 - 59	NS	-.09**	-.29***	-.12***
60 - 69	NS	-.12***	-.36***	-.19***
Social status	.16***	-.06*	.07**	NS
Chronic conditions	NS	.08**	.07**	NS
Social contacts	---	NS	---	NS
Group participation	---	NS	---	NS
Lack of supports	-.15***	.24***	.06*	NS
Life events stress	---	.20***	---	---
Locus of control				
Internal	-.09***	NS	-.05*	NS
Powerful others	NS	.06*	.06*	.09***
Chance	-.06**	.11***	NS	NS
Married	NS	NS	-.14***	-.14***
Employed	-.13***	NS	NS	---
Early loss of parent(s)	-.07**	NS	NS	NS

Note. Numbers are betas. Significance levels for groups are in relation to No-surgery, for time to the 12-15 month block, and for age to the 30-39 decade. For locus of control, higher scores indicate greater external control expectancies.

* $p < .05$, ** $p < .01$, *** $p < .001$, NS=not significant

Family Interaction Dysfunction

None of the study groups was distinguishable from each other on this measure of dysfunctional illness behavior in relation to family members (Tables 8 and 9). There was a time effect in the longitudinal component of the study of lessened disruption in relationships over time (Figure 2). Also, women in the older decades were less likely to report such occurrences.

In both study components, more dysfunctional interaction with family was predicted by life change stresses, poorer social supports and a locus of control in the direction of less personal control and more chance control over events. Also, lower social status and concurrent chronic medical conditions emerged as contributors to dysfunction in the cross-sectional analysis. Seventeen percent of the variation in reported dysfunctional behavior was explained by the variables in the regression equation.

Personal and Social Life Events Stress

The study groups were not significantly different from each other on this measure in either study component (Tables 8 and 9). The measure documents the impact of major personal decisions, achievements, troubles, losses and changes. Time and age effects were found; increasing age lessened the likelihood of such stresses for all groups in both study components as did time since surgery in the longitudinal component (Figure 2).

As a predictor in both study components, married women were significantly less likely to report such stresses. As a predictor in the regression analysis, higher social status increased the likelihood of such change stresses as did concurrent medical conditions, greater lack of social supports and greater belief in life outcomes as contingent on powerful others. However, those who assigned less responsibility to themselves for such outcomes decreased the likelihood of stress. The variables in the regression equation accounted for only nine percent of variation in life events stress.

Workplace Life Events Stress

Again, no group differences were found in either study component for this measure of work change readjustment; none of the study groups are distinguishable from the No-Surgery referent group

Table 9

Repeated Measures Analysis of Variance for Social Function Outcomes Showing Main Effects and Direction of Covariate Effects (Longitudinal Component).

	Social Health	Dysfunctional Interaction with Family	Personal and Social Life Events Stress	Workplace Life Events Stress	Social Role Functions Impairment	Daily Life Activities Impairment
Main Effects						
Group	NS	NS	NS	NS	$p < .05$	NS
Time	NS	$p < .001$	$p < .01$	NS	$p < .001$	$p < .01$
Group x Time	NS	NS	NS	$p < .05$	p .001	$p < .001$
Covariates						
Age 40 - 49	NS	-*	-***	NS	NS	NS
50 - 59	NS	-**	-***	-*	NS	NS
60 - 69	NS	-*	-***	-***	NS	NS
Social status	+*	NS	NS	NS	NS	NS
Chronic conditions	NS	NS	NS	NS	NS	NS
Lack of support	-***	+***	NS	NS	+***	+***
Life events stress	NS	+***	---	---	+***	+*
Locus of control	NS	+**	---	---	NS	+**
Married	NS	NS	-*	-*	NS	NS

Note. Significance levels for age are in relation to age decade 30-39. For locus of control, higher scores indicate external control.

* $p < .05$ ** $p < .01$. *** $p < .001$ NS=not significant

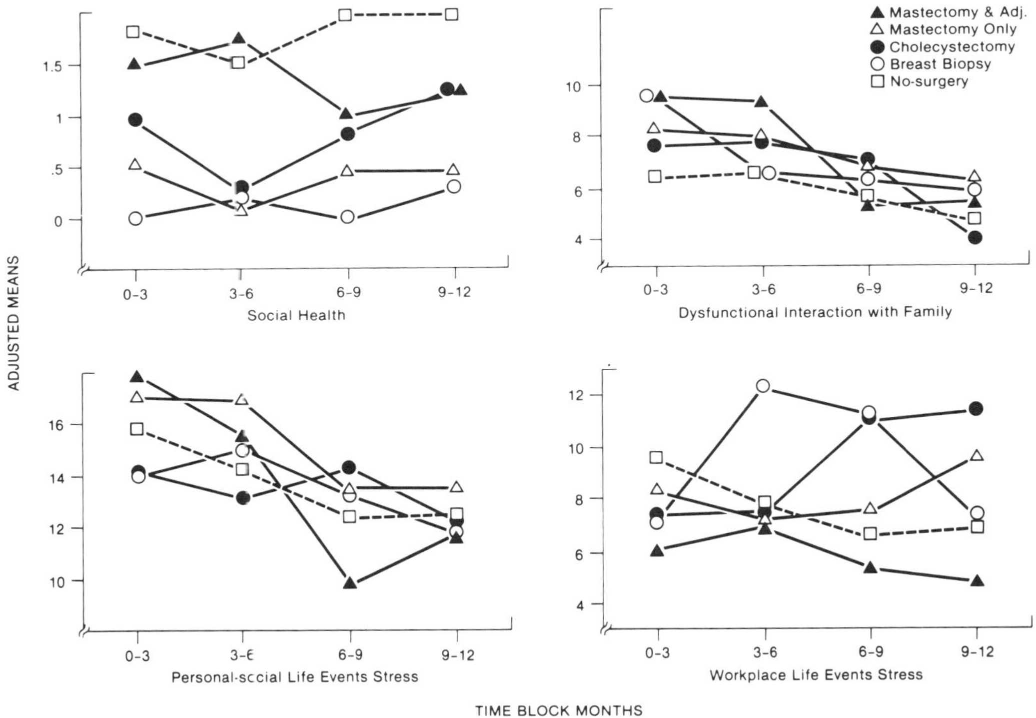

FIGURE 2. Mean scores, covariate adjusted, by time block for four social function outcomes (longitudinal component).

(Tables 8 and 9, Figure 2). Women over fifty and married women, both groups with lower employment, reported correspondingly less workplace change. Of the remaining predictor variables, locus of control, entered only into the cross-sectional analysis, was significant and only four percent of the variance in that equation was explained by the study variables.

Social Role Impairment

Both of the Mastectomy groups showed evidence of more impairment in their social role functions than the referent No-Surgery group on this interviewer rating made at the first and fourth assessment periods in the longitudinal study component only (Table 9). There was no age effect in this measure but there was a time effect. The group differences observed in the 0–3 months time block disappeared by the 0–12 months assessment (Figure 3).

Life events stress and perceived lack of emotional support were significant predictors of role impairment across groups.

Daily Life Activities Impairment

Statistically significant group differences were not found for this interviewer rating completed at the 0–3 months and 9–12 months assessments (Table 9, Figure 3). Again, age effects were not observed, but time effects were observed. There was a decrease in impairment for all surgical groups over the elapsed time.

Predictors of impairment in activities and involvements of daily life were life-change stresses, lack of emotional support and a less internally oriented locus of control expectancy.

DISCUSSION

These findings provide only very limited support for our main study hypothesis that on each of the ten indicators selected as outcome measures of psychosocial function, the mastectomy groups would show a measurable and significant difference in the direction of poorer outcome from the No-Surgery group which would be greater than that of the surgical comparison groups. We found significant group differences for only four of the ten psychosocial

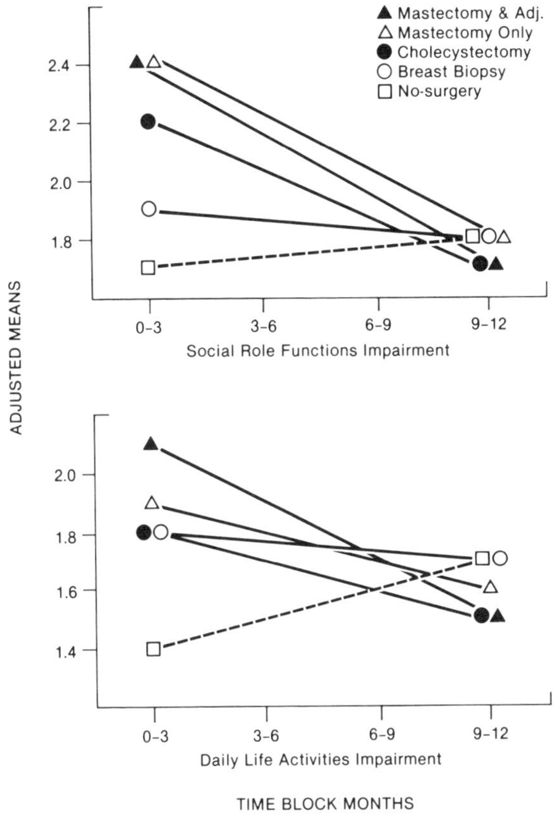

FIGURE 3. Mean scores, covariate adjusted, by time block for two social function outcomes (longitudinal component).

outcomes chosen for study. There were differences in body image dissatisfaction and feminine self-image concerns which were confined to the mastectomy group treated by mastectomy alone. Further, these differences, although significant, were small and accounted for very little of the total variance observed in the respective outcome measures.

A difference in social health evidenced by the group treated by mastectomy alone did not extend to the mastectomy group receiving adjuvant therapy and was also shared with other surgical groups. The only further evidence of the impact of mastectomy was that both mastectomy groups had more difficulty initially in carrying out expected social role functions than the non-surgical comparison group. However, the difference in function was small and not distinguishable from that of the cholecystectomy group.

The findings from the longitudinal study reinforced those from the cross-sectional study, giving increased support to the results reported.

In considering the results of this study, it is important to keep in mind that the study selection criteria precluded pre-existing serious mental or physical disability. Within this previously healthy sample then, we found that women treated by mastectomy alone for breast cancer did not, as a group, report measurable disability in the self-concept or social aspects of their lives that could not be attributed to the impact of a surgical procedure per se. The women who received adjuvant therapy in addition to mastectomy as a group did report a measurably poorer outcome in feminine self-image and body image compared to all other groups, but the difference was not greatly divergent from them.

Our findings challenge the assumption that breast surgery automatically results in an increased incidence of psychosocial disability. Rather, women, at least between the ages of 30 to 69 and without pre-existing serious mental or physical problems, were able to use their coping resources to make a successful psychosocial adaptation. Our results are similar to those of earlier surveys which reported overall a good quality of survival among mastectomy patients (Craig, Comstock and Geiser, 1974; Eisenberg and Goldenberg, 1966; and Schottenfeld and Robbins, 1970). Adaptation may have been easier for the women in our study than in earlier decades because of the increased information about cancer available to the general public, the reduction of stigma attached to cancer as a disease, the generally greater acceptance by the treatment community of women's rights to participate in treatment decisions, the trend toward less radical surgical procedures, increasing opportunities for breast reconstruction, the widespread availability of the Reach to Recovery Program and a growing number of hospital support groups, and the increasing awareness of the importance of psychosocial factors by caregivers in oncology settings. Forty-four percent of the mastectomy group in our study had biopsy and mastectomy in separate stages indicating an increased opportunity for information about treatment options and advance psychological preparation that might not have been the case even a decade earlier. We did not record whether mastectomy patients in our study had been offered future breast reconstruction or whether they received post-mastectomy counseling from health professionals or volunteers, so we cannot report on the benefit such factors might have played in the adjustment process. No participants in the study were observed to be psychiatrically impaired to a degree that intervention of an emergency nature was required.

While the present study confined itself to observation of women without pre-existing serious mental or physical illness, it might be assumed that women who had such conditions would be more vulnerable to poorer outcome.

Additionally, our study does not address outcomes for women over the age of 69, and half of all breast cancer patients are over the age of 65. Where age differences were observed in our study, they showed uniformly more favorable psychosocial outcomes with increasing age. The interpretation of these findings can only be speculated upon and whether they would carry through to even older decades is not apparent. The concerns of older women may be tempered by experience and perspective and their concerns may also be different from those of younger women. On the other hand, the increased physical frailty and greater likelihood of more concurrent medical conditions may render some aspects of adaptation more difficult for individuals more elderly than we studied.

While the resilience of body self-concept after mastectomy has been noted (Weinstein, Vetter and Serson, 1967), other authors have suggested that for mastectomy patients there is a period of denial about body image and feminine self-image which serves as a necessary defense during recovery and that reactions to cancer surgery and breast loss may be delayed until several months after surgery or longer. Polivy (1977) observed a decline in body image of mastectomy patients six to ten months after surgery. While no such obvious pattern for body image was observed in our data, denial might partly account for the decreased reporting of feminine self-image concerns during the first post-surgical assessment period and for the differences in both body image and feminine self-image between the two mastectomy groups in our study. In addition to such tangible changes as hair loss due to chemotherapy or skin discoloration from radiotherapy, the women receiving adjuvant therapies may have been less able to sustain denial in the face of ongoing medical treatments and potentially more serious disease. Adjuvant treatment itself gives rise to impairment in sexual relationships for some women. For example, Meyerowitz, Sparks and Spears (1979) reported an adverse effect of adjuvant chemotherapy for breast cancer on marital and sexual relationships of women they studied, with life disruptions increasing until treatment was stopped, and Silverfarb, Maurer and Crouthamel (1980) reported disturbance in mate role, primarily lessened sexual desire by women during active treatment by radiotherapy and chemotherapy for primary breast cancer.

The hypotheses concerning the predictor variables chosen for examination in our study were generally confirmed. Where they emerged as significant predictors they performed in the hypothesized direction (with the exception of employment) and were often better predictors of psychosocial outcome than surgical group membership. Social contacts per se did not emerge as a predictor of psychosocial outcomes. More important as a predictor for nearly all outcomes selected was the measure of social support used, which rather than documenting patterns of social affiliation such as frequency and extent of social contacts with family or friends, served as an index of individuals' perceptions or expectations that comfort, concern, advice, positive or affectionate regard, help with problems and the like would be available from those close to them. This finding buttresses Cobb's (1976) emphasis on perceived social support, one of the many measures of social support which have been put forward for study (Bloom, 1978; Murawski, Penman and Schmitt, 1978), which is particularly relevant here because fear about withdrawal of support by significant others is cited as common among post-mastectomy concerns. Among other predictors, the most important across psychosocial outcomes were chronic medical conditions, the stress of life events and locus of control expectancy. Thus the context in which the surgical event occurs is of importance as is the individual's emotional disposition.

The predictors suggest that post-mastectomy women vulnerable to poorer outcome would be those with other pre-existing chronic diseases, lower expectations of good quality social support, other present life stressors, and a disposition to believe in life outcomes as less under their own control and more contingent on the authority or influence of others, findings parallel to those of Worden and Weisman (1977). For such individuals, adaptation may best be facilitated by interventions such as those described by Bloom, Ross and Burnell (1978), which attempt to increase women's sense of personal efficacy and control, suggested as particularily important by Taylor and Levin (1976b) and others, and provide a counseling or peer support group experience which is accepting, sympathetic to the women's particular experience, does not minimize the very real adaptation required and is supportive to that effort.

REFERENCES

Berscheid, E., Walster, E., and Bohrnstedt, G., (1972). Body Image: A Psychology Today questionnaire. *Psychology Today*, *6*, 58–66.

Bloom, J.R. (1978, September). *Social support systems and cancer: A conceptual view.* Paper presented to the Psychosocial Study Group, California Division of the American Cancer Society, Coronado, CA.

Bloom, J.R., Ross, R.D., and Burnell, G. (1978). The effects of social support on patient adjustment after breast surgery. *Patient Counseling and Health Education*, *1* (2), 50–59.

Cobb, S. (1976). Social support as a moderator of life stress, *Psychosomatic Medicine*, *38* (5), 300–314.

Craig, T.J., Comstock, G.W., and Geiser, P.B. (1974). The quality of survival in breast cancer: A case-control comparison. *Cancer*, *33*, 1451–1457.

Donald, C.A., and Ware, J.E. (1982). *Quantification of Social Contacts and Resources.* (Publication No. R-2937-HHS). Santa Monica: Rand Corporation.

Eisenberg, H.S., and Goldenberg, I.S. (1966). A measurement of quality of survival of breast cancer patients. In J.L. Hayward and R.D. Bulbrook (Eds.), *Clinical evaluation of breast cancer* (pp. 93–108). London: Academic Press.

Flamer, D. (1977). *Perception of Social Support.* Unpublished manuscript. (Available from the author, Shaklee Corp., 444 Market St., San Francisco, CA).

Gilson, B.S., Gilson, J.S., Bergner, M. et al. (1975). The sickness impact profile: Development of an outcome measure of health care. *American Journal of Public Health*, *65* (12), 1304–10.

Hollingshead, A.G. *Four factor index of social status (a working paper).* Unpublished manuscript, Yale University, New Haven.

Holmes, T.H., and Rahe, R.H. (1967). The social readjustment rating scale. *Journal of Psychosomatic research*, *11*, 213–218.

Levenson, H. (1974). Activism and powerful others: Distinctions within the concept of internal-external control. *Journal of Personality Assessment*, *38* (4), 377–383.

Lewis, F.M., and Bloom, J.R. (1978–79). Psychosocial adjustment to breast cancer: A review of selected literature. *International Journal of Psychiatry in Medicine*, *9* (11), 1–17.

Meyerowitz, B.E. (1980). Psychosocial correlates of breast cancer and its treatments. *Psychological Bulletin*, *87* (1) 108–131

Meyerowitz, B.E., Sparkes, F.C., and Spears, I.K. (1979). Psychosocial impact of adjuvant chemotherapy for breast carcinoma. *Cancer*, *43*, 1613–8.

Murawski, B.J., Penman, D., and Schmitt, M. (1978). Social support in health and illness: The concept and its measurement. *Cancer Nursing*, *1*, 365–371.

National Cancer Institute (1978). *Psychological aspects of breast cancer: An annotated bibliography relevant to intervention design.* (DHEW publication No. NIH78-1550). Washington, DC: U.S. Government Printing Office.

Polivy, J. (1977). Psychological effects of mastectomy on a woman's feminine self-concept. *Journal of Nervous and Mental Disease*, *164* (2), 77–86.

Rosenberg, M. (1965). *Society and the adolescent self-image.* Princeton: Princeton University Press.

Schain, W. (1977). *Personal Problem Checklist.* Unpublished manuscript. (Available from the author, 5335 Strathmore Ave., Kensington, MD).

Schottenfeld, D., and Robbins, G. (1970). Quality of survival among patients who have had radical mastectomy. *Cancer*, *26*, 650–655.

Silverfarb, P.M., Maurer, L.H., and Crouthamel, C.S. (1980). Psychosocial aspects of neoplastic disease: I. Functional status of breast cancer patients during different treatment regimens. *American Journal of Psychiatry*, *137* (4), 450–455.

Spitzer, R.L., Endicott, J., Mesnikoff, A.M., and Cohen, G.M. (1968). *Psychiatric evaluation form*. New York: Biometrics Research, New York State Department of Mental Hygiene, New York State Psychiatric Institute.

Taylor, S.E., and Levin, S. (1976a). *Psychological aspects of breast cancer: A conceptual overview of the literature and annotated bibliography*. San Francisco: West Coast Cancer Foundation.

Taylor, S.E., and Levin, S. (1976b). *The psychological impact of breast cancer: A review of theory and research*. San Francisco: West Coast Cancer Foundation.

Ware, J.E. (1976). *The conceptualization and measurement of health for policy relevant research in medical care delivery*. Paper presented at the meeting of the American Association for the Advancement of Science, Boston, MA.

Weinstein, S., Vetter, R.J., and Serson, E.A. (1967). Preferences for bodily parts following mastectomy. *American Journal of Psychology*, *80*, (458–461).

Worden, J.W., and Weisman, A. (1977). The fallacy in postmastectomy depression. *American Journal of the Medical Sciences*, *273*, 169–175.

Laryngectomy Rehabilitation: A Woman's Viewpoint

Grace F. Ulbricht

ABSTRACT. A laryngectomy can be a traumatic operation, emotionally as well as physically. A female laryngectomee describes the emotional and physical problems that women face following this operation, especially in dealing with the complete and permanent loss of speech, and in managing a disfiguring stoma in the neck area. Support of family and friends, assistance of an experienced speech pathologist, and guidance from other caring health professionals all play a vital role in helping the laryngectomee master esophageal speech and begin once again to lead a full, productive life.

Cancer of the larynx has often been thought of as a "man's disease" because the incidence is more than six times as great in men as in women. This still means, however, that of the 11,700 new cases predicted for 1986 by the American Cancer Society, about 2,100 will be in women. About 60% of these women will require surgical removal of the larynx, an operation called a laryngectomy. A person who undergoes this operation is called a laryngectomee.

The primary concern of this paper is the impact of this surgery on women and their special needs for total rehabilitation. All laryngectomees have similar problems, but women encounter certain difficulties and prejudices which do not appear to affect their male counterparts with the same severity.

A laryngectomy is a traumatic experience. It causes a disability which has a psychological and social impact of devastating proportions. It causes the immediate loss of vocal sounds of any kind and the permanent loss of the natural voice. It causes the immediate impairment of the senses of taste and smell, which are never fully restored, and for the rest of the patient's life the only way she will

Grace F. Ulbricht recently retired as Director of Consumer Relations, F.W. Woolworth Co.

breathe, cough, or sneeze is through the unsightly opening just above the base of the neck.

This surgery, coming so soon after the initial shock of learning one has cancer, can prove to be more than the patient can handle. However, it has been found that if she was reasonably well adjusted before surgery, if her illness and the surgery were properly explained by the surgeon, and, most importantly, she has the love and support of her spouse, family, and friends, the patient will emerge in the same sound mental state.

Fifteen years ago I had a total laryngectomy and radical neck dissection. I was lucky. I had a caring surgeon, a loving family, and supportive friends. I mastered esophageal speech. I lived. In the ensuing years I have found there is a lack of knowledge and understanding among health care professionals of the problems encountered by laryngectomees.

Doctors do, of course, know what a laryngectomy is. However, lacking recent experience with the surgery, some have forgotten a few important aspects. To illustrate, I was in a major metropolitan hospital last year for openheart surgery. The examining physician, who knew I was a laryngectomee, told me to take a deep breath through my mouth. I opened my mouth and took a deep breath through my stoma. He never noticed the difference.

I am not a professional in the health-care field and am in no way qualified to comment on surgical procedures. It is the prerogative of the doctor to determine what, if any, voice prostheses should be considered, or if the patient should be able to learn esophageal speech. I can, however, give an overview of the physical and emotional problems faced by a laryngectomee, in particular, one who is a woman.

The first several days are filled with pain in the throat area and, if the patient had neck surgery on one or both sides, she will ache from the ear down through the shoulder and arm. The resulting shoulder freeze can all but make the arm immobile. To some degree the ache can last for a number of years.

Food is denied for several days and she is fed intravenously and through a tube inserted in the nose, through the pharnyx and esophagus, and into the stomach. She will be given soft food as soon as the throat area has healed sufficiently. It can be a number of weeks before regular food is allowed.

Breathing is completely different. Air no longer circulates from the lungs to the nose and mouth, but through the stoma, now the only air passage to the lungs. Mucus collects in the lungs and exits through the stoma, which must be kept clear at all times. A laryngectomee will have mucus for the rest of her life, but immediately following surgery it is excessive. This mucus crusts around the edge of the stoma and must be wiped away to avoid irritation and odor. A tube is inserted in the stoma to keep it open. This is usually removed after a few weeks, although some patients need it the rest of their lives.

In addition to the mucus, there is a great deal of coughing. In time this diminishes. However, throughout her lifetime a laryngectomee will be troubled by small particles of dust or air pollution which irritate the passageway to the lungs and cause coughing and more mucus.

After the first day or two of dealing with all these new problems, the patient becomes aware of the fact that she cannot make any vocal sounds. Following major surgery, every patient cries. When a laryngectomee cries, there may be floods of tears, but there is complete silence. The body shakes with sobs, but there is no sound. When this fact is realized it can be shattering.

During a patient's hospitalization, she is watched over and cared for by experienced nurses and technicians. Her surgeon visits regularly, checking on her progress. She is warm and safe. Once discharged, she is on her own. In the outside world the true terror of the situation sets in.

The first look in the mirror is devastating. The stoma is located at the base of the neck. It is open and obvious. If there has been additional neck surgery, that side of the neck is sunken and forever after will have a "scrawny" appearance. The immediate problem is to cover the disfigurement and at the same time allow air to get into the lungs. A man can place a piece of gauze over the stoma, put on a shirt and tie and go about his business. A woman, because most dresses are open at the neckline, must devise attractive measures to cover the stoma. Until this problem is solved, she may find herself a virtual prisoner in her home.

Once covered, the stoma is not forgotten. It is especially difficult for a woman to learn to accept this permanent disfigurement. The neck is a sensitive, sensuous area of the body and important in love making. After surgery some women cannot imagine any man wanting to stroke or kiss her mutilated neck.

All laryngectomees must learn to manage the stoma. Once more, because of the mode of dress, women have greater problems than men. We never know when we will experience irritants in the air which cause coughing and mucus discharge. This discharge is the problem. If not checked in time, it runs down the chest. If that area is not covered, the mucus is visible.

Everything about a laryngectomy is unfeminine. The most obvious is the sound of the new voice. I was able to master esophageal speech, but it took over a year before I could be understood. The pitch of esophageal speech is at least an octave lower than laryngeal speech. Subconsciously many women find this so objectionable they cannot learn alaryngeal speech and even refuse to use an electronic speech aid. In a highly emotional situation, laryngectomees cannot make a sound. We can never make the sounds of crying, shouting, or of laughter. We have lost most of that type of self-expression, which loss adds to our frustrations. We feel the limitations and penalties caused by our surgery.

Any surgery which leaves permanent disfigurement or scarring can affect the way we think, feel and act. Combined with the stoma problems and the strange new sounds of attempted speech, a woman can feel completely defeated and no longer feminine. Recovering our feeling of femininity can be a serious problem. One of the special joys of being a woman is the pleasure in wearing a feminine scent, a perfume that tells the wearer and those around her that she is a woman. Now perfume can irritate the passageway to the lungs and cause coughing. Also, since we no longer breathe through the nose, our sense of smell has diminished.

Usually, cancer of the larynx occurs into and beyond middle age. Consequently, most female laryngectomees were children when girls were girls and boys a privileged breed apart; well before women were "liberated." When we were small, girls were taught to rely on men and not on themselves. This feeling of dependency, or inferiority, was ingrained. Now, following a laryngectomy some women find themselves turning inward and becoming consumed with worry that since they have had cancer, resulting in this terrible surgery, they are no longer good enough to keep the love of husband and family. Some women require special counseling for this feeling of inadequacy. Not all husbands are supportive. Women have great capacity to love, and overlook any imperfections in their husbands. Unfortunately, not all men or women can do this, and some marriages dissolve.

It is evident that female laryngectomees need many different kinds of physical and emotional support in special ways. Fortunately, these kinds of help are available for all laryngectomees. Ideally, the surgeon should direct his patient to the proper source, but experience has shown this is not always the case. It has been the experience of many of my fellow laryngectomees that following successful surgery the surgeon has little or no interest in the rehabilitation of his patients, male or female. He simply refers them to a speech pathologist.

An informed, caring surgeon will contact the local unit of the American Cancer Society asking that a laryngectomee with good alaryngeal speech visit his patient both before and after surgery. This patient/visitor relationship is vital to ensure the well being of each new patient during the transitional period between silence and speech. He will also ask the hospital or the ACS to arrange for a social worker to visit his patient. Other than that, there seems to be no formal follow-up of a patient's speech progress by the medical profession.

The ACS sponsors the International Association of Laryngectomees (IAL) and member clubs of the IAL are located in nearly all 50 states, the District of Columbia and many foreign countries. It is mostly through these support groups that laryngectomees, both new and oldtimers, are given any information and continuing help they need.

In the past, most laryngectomees received alaryngeal speech training at a member club. This was free of charge and conducted by members who had undergone similar surgery, were emotionally well adjusted, and had good alaryngeal speech. Recently, however, more than 30 state governments have passed a licensure law making it illegal for persons not licensed to teach laryngectomees alarygeal speech, except under direct supervision of a speech pathologist. This has made it difficult for some new laryngectomees who lack funds, do not have insurance, and are not qualified for financial aid. It is also a fact that in some areas of the country there are few, if any, speech pathologists skilled in teaching alaryngeal speech.

The laryngectomee clubs are, however, alive and well. Although many are no longer permitted to teach speech, they do hold regular meetings where all phases of rehabilitation are discussed and demonstrated. The IAL holds an annual convention in various sections of the country which all laryngectomees, and those interested in laryngectomee rehabilitation, are welcome to attend. Free lessons by speech pathologists are provided during the four-day convention and the IAL Voice Institute is held the week preceding the convention.

This Institute provides instruction in alaryngeal speech for laryngectomees and teaching instruction for speech pathologists and qualified laryngectomees with good alaryngeal speech.

I do not intend to leave my readers with negative feelings. There is life after laryngectomy and one of the most rewarding aspects of this new life with a new voice is the personal satisfaction one finds learning to speak, overcoming any handicaps, and helping those who follow. Had I not been a laryngectomee I would not have been invited to Tokyo, Japan, to speak at the Third World Congress of Laryngectomees, or to Barcelona, Spain, to address the 32nd International Congress of Laryngectomees. Please encourage new laryngectomees as they come to your attention. They are not alone and with proper guidance, emotional support and teaching, they will find a bright new world of adventure theirs for the taking.

Female Cancer Patients and Caregivers: Experiences in the Workplace

Frances Lomas Feldman, PhD

ABSTRACT. Working women who have a cancer history, or who have some responsibility for the care of relatives with cancer, often face a cluster of attitudes and behaviors in their employers and co-workers to which individuals touched by other kinds of illness are not exposed. Patients and caregivers may find that others in the work environment are compassionate and helpful in many ways, but may also encounter considerable hostility and fear expressed verbally or as shunning or other attitudinal problems in the worksite. They may also be targets of overt or covert discrimination. These problems are explored using data from three recent studies on workplace experiences of white collar and blue collar workers who had recovered from cancer, and of former pediatric cancer patients.

THE IMPACT OF CANCER

Whatever reasons motivate her to enter the labor force, a woman's working role tends to define her in our society as a work-oriented, productive, and independent person, and it often contributes to her self-perceptions as responsible, autonomous, and mistress of her own destiny. In essence, she incorporates the societal attitudes that equate work with adequacy, independence and worthiness.

To the work-oriented individual, work performance may symbolize continued mastery over one's own future, confidence in one's own integrity as an individual, and a defense against abysmal depression. Following cancer, involuntary job loss or deterioration of conditions under which the work is performed can produce stress inimical to a woman's physical and mental well-being. The life-threatening nature of cancer often evokes in the patient and others an almost overwhelming picture of inexorable pain and imminent

Frances Lomas Feldman is Professor Emerita, School of Social Work, University of Southern California, Los Angeles, CA 90007.

death. Her anger and fear may be reinforced by the mournful demeanor and a cluster of other attitudes about cancer expressed by associates and relatives, giving rise to a sense of hopelessness and helplessness about control over the cancer and, by extension, over the quality and duration of the individual's life. If other life-crisis events occur as a consequence of or coincident with the cancer diagnosis (in the marriage or other personal relationships, or in connection with financial or work security), there is further diminution of autonomy over self.

But cancer is not necessarily a fatal disease, and many women return to the workplace after they are treated or cured. It is to work performance that the victim of cancer can elect to arrogate attributes of self-management, independence of spirit, and value as a human being; the work role offers the individual whose life is jeopardized by illness a tactile and visible battleground.

Over a period of time, the California Division of the American Cancer Society received a number of written and verbal communications protesting discriminatory practices in the workplace against recovered cancer patients. A clinical analysis of these (McKenna, 1973) led the Division to sponsor a trilogy of successive studies to learn the nature of work experiences, positive as well as negative, of individuals with a cancer history. The aim was to gather data that might provide guidelines for action regarding patients' service needs, public policy considerations, and public and professional education (Feldman, 1976; 1978; 1980). The McKenna subjects were self-selected. Two other studies compared post-cancer performance of employees with performance of other employees in the same organizations, finding no significant differences (Wheatley, 1972; Stone, 1975).

The Trilogy of Work and Cancer Studies

The objectives of the three studies were the same: (1) to describe the nature of workplace experiences of individuals able to return to work following a diagnosis of cancer; (2) to learn if the experiences, positive or negative, seemed connected with the cancer diagnosis or treatment and if patient-perceptions about negative associations with cancer could be corroborated; and (3) to assess how the work experiences, whatever their nature as perceived by the patient, affected the individual's quality of life.

The first study (WC) focused on white collar occupations,

nursing and teaching, while the second study (BC) drew its sample from blue collar and service occupations. Because survival rates among those with pediatric cancer now suggest many will have to become economically self-sufficient as adults, the third study (YS) looked not only at work experiences of young people but also at school experiences to discern elements that might influence the young patient's vocational expectation.

To optimize comparability, the three study designs were similar; several components were added to the BC and YC studies, suggested by the data that emerged from the WC inquiry. For example, data from subjects' doctors were collected in the second and third studies to learn what and how information was given to inquiring or prospective employers about diagnosis and prognosis; a sample of union officials was interviewed in the second study. Except for occupation, characteristics for inclusion of patients in the WC and BC studies were the same: fully employed at time of diagnosis (to demonstrate actual attachment to the work force); between the ages of 23 and 50 years at diagnosis (to reduce possibility of disqualification for work by reason of being too young or inexperienced, or too close to retirement age); cancer sites of head/neck, rectum/colon, or breast (because of high incidence and favorable survival rates). The YS sample was constructed to include youth diagnosed between the ages of 13 and 23 regardless of cancer site. This wide age range was chosen because it spans various developmental stages of adolescence.

The time elapsed between diagnosis and interview was restricted to between one and five years to put the diagnosis far enough in the past to allow time for the patient to resume or locate work. The adults were interviewed from one to two and a half years following diagnosis (median 2 years, 4 months); the youths were interviewed from one to five years after diagnosis (median 3 years, 8 months). A total of 344 patients were interviewed. Each study included interviews with doctors and with actual and potential employers. Parents and school personnel were interviewed in the YS study and, as already noted, unions in the BC study. In addition, all work experiences or work-seeking efforts reported by 12 patients in each study were tracked in order to ascertain congruence of patient and employer perceptions; from one to six such patient-reported experiences were followed. In like manner, school experiences were traced for some student-respondents.

Sources of Data Specific to Women

Not all the information contained in the three studies had been statistically analyzed by sex. However, for purposes of this article, the interview data in the trilogy were reviewed for incidents and trends among female patient-respondents as well as among female family members in the labor force who had some caregiving responsibility for any respondent in the patient samples; some were YS parents, others were spouses or other relatives who had participated in WC or BC patient-interviews or had sought out the research interviewers before or after the interview with the patient. The thrust of this reexamination was qualitative in nature and statistical tests were not made. In large measure, the content of this article derives from this reexamination, complemented by material subsequently obtained from formal and informal inquiries conducted by the author with individuals and groups. The nature and implications of some of the work experiences of the work-able woman cancer patient will be addressed first, then experiences of working women who have certain responsibilities for family members with cancer.

WORK EXPERIENCES OF THE RECOVERED WOMAN CANCER PATIENT

Interviews were held with 229 women patients (67 percent of all the subjects): 98 (71%) of the 138 WC patients; 86 (70%) of the 123 BC respondents; and 45 (54%) of the 83 YS respondents. Some selected characteristics of these interviewees are presented in Table 1; Table 2 shows their distribution by cancer site.

While all the female respondents were under age 50 at diagnosis, a fourth of the WC and BC women had passed this age by the time of interview; 29 percent still were under 45 years. The age balance also had shifted among the YS respondents: from more than half under 18 years at diagnosis to more than half (55 percent) over 18 and already in or trying to enter the labor force.

How had these youthful and adult respondents fared with respect to attachment to the work force? At diagnosis, all the WC and BC respondents had been fully employed. At interview, they regarded themselves as employable although, as Table 3 shows, approximately a fourth of the WC and just over a third of the BC women either were working only part time or not at all. Among the latter

TABLE 1

Selected Characteristics of Female Patient-Respondents by Study
(Percentages in Parentheses)

Study:	WC	BC	YS	Total
No. of subjects:	98	86	45	229
AGE AT DIAGNOSIS				
45 - 50 yr	61 (62)	58 (67)		119 (52)
23 - 45 yr	37 (38)	28 (33)		65 (28)
18 - 23 yr			22 (49)	22 (10)
under 18 yr			23 (51)	23 (10)
LIVING ARRANGEMENTS				
At Diagnosis:				
Married, with spouse	70 (71)[a]	65 (76)[a]	11 (24)	
Unmarried, with parents			32 (71)	
Living alone	28 (29)	21 (24)	2 (4)	
At Interview:				
Married, with spouse	66 (67)[a]	64 (74)[a]	18 (40)[b]	
Unmarried, with parents			13 (29)[c]	
Living alone	28 (29)	7 (8)	14 (31)	
Living with unrelated adults	4 (4)	15 (17)		

[a] Includes some marriages or remarriage subsequent to diagnosis, as well as dissolution of marriages by divorce or death.

[b] Five married couples moved into parental homes after diagnosis.

[c] Two had lived alone but returned to parental home after diagnosis.

Abbreviations: WC = White Collar Study. BC = Blue Collar Study. YS = Youth-Student Study

were four who had elected to retire along with their newly-retired husbands. Except for four of the not-employed and four of the partly-employed, the other unemployed and partly unemployed women felt able and ready for full time employment. More than half of the YS females were students only at time of diagnosis. As Table 3 shows, this picture had altered by interview: the proportion of respondents attached to the labor force had increased—in part a function of age and completion of education; nearly a third (31 percent) had unsuccessfully been seeking work.

To learn how the cancer health history affected the employable adult or youthful respondents in relation to procuring or retaining a place in the work force, the Work and Cancer Histories studies had queried patients first about their pre-cancer health, work preparation, and experience; then they were asked about their expectations

TABLE 2

Female Patient-Respondents, by Cancer Site and Study
(Percentages in Parentheses)

Study:	WC	BC	YS	Total
No. of subjects:	98	86	45	229
CANCER SITE				
Head and neck	21 (21)	11 (13)		32 (14)
Colon and Rectum	25 (26)	27 (31)		52 (23)
Breast	52 (53)	48 (56)		100 (44)
Hodgkins			17 (38)	17 (7)
Leukemia			6 (13)	6 (3)
Bones and soft tissues			6 (13)	6 (3)
Thyroid			12 (27)	12 (5)
Other			4 (9)	4 (2)

Abbreviations: WC = White Collar Study. BC = Blue Collar Study.
YS = Youth-Student Study

TABLE 3

Work Status of Women Patients at Time of Diagnosis
and at Time of Interview

(Percentages in Parentheses)

Study:	WC		BC		YS	
No. of subjects:	98		86		45	
	At DX	At Interview	At DX	At Interview	At DX	At Interview
Working full time	98 (100)	74 (76)	86 (100)	57 (66)	11 (25)	27 (60)
Working part time		13 (13)		16 (19)	8 (18)	3 (7)
Unemployed, seeking work		11 (11)		13 (15)		15 (33)
Full time students only					26 (57)	11 (25)
In school and working						16 (36)
Neither in school nor working						3 (6)
Working for pre-cancer employer		70 (71)		53 (62)		14 (31)
Looking for some or other work because of cancer		28 (29)		33 (38)		14 (31)

Abbreviations: WC = White Collar Study. BC = Blue Collar Study.
YS = Youth-Student Study

and actual experiences on return to work. The focus was on tasks, organizations, associates, health, and other relevant elements that could provide a "before and after" view of the individual in the work place.

Positive Work Place Experiences

Nearly two-thirds of all the respondents reported positive experiences in their work life after the diagnosis. Fellow workers as well as employers were helpful in many ways. Patients were relieved of some tasks until physical strength could be restored. A waitress in a "topless" bar, for example, had secretly delayed for nearly a year in consulting a doctor about a lump on her breast, fearful she would lose her breast *and* job and not find other work of the only kind she had ever done. Her employer not only designed a special costume for her, but assigned a bus boy to carry her trays until she could comfortably raise her arms above her shoulders. The work schedules of many were unquestioningly adjusted to accommodate medical treatment. Some reported alteration in equipment to aid the patients' management of work assignments: telephone equipment was changed to facilitate use by women with artificial voice boxes (see paper by Ulbricht elsewhere in this issue); an assembly line rotation was changed so the patient could leave the line as needed without affecting the assembly operations.

The positive behavior of others in the worksite was sometimes perceived by the patient as remarkable, the more so when the patient had fearfully expected to be the direct target of negative reactions. One middle-aged executive secretary to the corporation president had held her position for only six months when unanticipated surgery resulted in severe facial disfigurement. Certain she had lost this job, that her age combined with her appearance precluded finding *anything*, and that her working life was over, she was deeply depressed. Visiting her in the hosptial, her boss "demanded" she stop "feeling sorry" for herself and hurry back to work. She did. Her continued productivity led to advances in salary and responsibilities, including face to face meetings with important clients.

Cancer-Related Work Problems

Yet even women who described some associates in the work environment as helpful or compassionate or who treated them as though "nothing had happened," frequently attributed work problems to how others felt about working near or with someone with cancer. More than half of the WC women, more than 80 percent of the BC women, and more than half of the YS girls and women, whether in the labor force or students, ascribed problems to how others reacted to the cancer history. Following the cancer diagnosis, 80 percent of the women sought to change their employment. Some stated that new awareness of their mortality led them to look for more self-fulfilling work or work schedules that could more readily enable them to pursue personal and family interests that held new attractions for them. Others wanted to advance themselves, with cancer merely a propelling force for action they had contemplated prior to the illness. But the majority were motivated by "discriminatory" or "unfair" conditions they attributed to reactions seemingly provoked in others by the cancer history. These reactions were manifest in negative changes in employee benefits or working conditions, unpleasant undertones or outright hostility among one or more fellow workers or superiors.

By interview, many of these women had abandoned efforts to effect a job change. Some were discouraged by repeated rejections they blamed on bias or lack of understanding about cancer. Some feared they might be excluded from health and other benefits because of their pre-existing medical condition. The wish to change, even when the patient made no attempt to implement it, perhaps is even more significant in view of the long seniority of these employees in the pre-cancer job: more than half of the BC and WC women (54 percent) had been with that employer for more than ten years, only 11 percent for a year or less. Among the 19 YS female respondents with full or part time work at diagnosis, nearly one-third returned to the pre-cancer employer and an equal proportion of these subsequently tried to find other employment because of problems they associated with the cancer diagnosis or treatment. Outcomes of these efforts were evenly divided among those who did and did not find other work.

Yet all three studies contained some respondents who had changed jobs not just through their own searches, but on invitation initiated by the new employers. Some of the latter knew the patient had serious problems in the pre-cancer work situation; others had no knowledge at all of the cancer history.

Categories of Cancer-Related Work Problems

Three categories of work problems were identified without regard for whether they were labeled by the patient as "prejudice," "discrimination," or other pejorative terminology. *Gross discrimination* included dismissal or demotion; denial of promotion or of a job or cost-of-living or other upward wage adjustment accorded other employees; termination or reduction or exclusion from health or life or retirement benefits; or undesired modification of other work conditions, with the cancer experience specified as the reason. Examples are the teacher reassigned from classroom teaching after a mastectomy so the children would not be "exposed" to her, and the nurse with cancer of the thyroid who was transferred to night duty to reduce the number of fellow workers (not patients!) who would have contact with her. Both of these instances were confirmed by third-party interviews.

A second category of work problems centered on attitudes encountered in the work environment that did not necessarily lead to changes in hours, wages or salaries, benefits, job retention, or other working conditions, but resembled strongly the precipitating attitudinal circumstances and responses found in the gross discrimination group. These *workplace attitudes* included ostracism by fellow workers and/or superiors and/or subordinates; overt hostility, like mimicry of the individual using an artificial voice device, or confrontation of the patient in the women's rest room with "How does it feel to be less than a whole woman?" following a mastectomy; complaints by supervisors that patients "leaning too much" on others were "not worth their salt" even though neither quantity nor quality of their productivity had lessened and there was "clear" evidence that their performance at least equaled that of coworkers. Also classed among negative workplace attitudes were situations where the patients were unable to cope with the overly solicitous or protective behavior they found "smothering." These women complained that the unwanted "saccharin" attention diverted the patient's physical and emotional energies from the tasks at hand or that it implied the work able person no longer was capable of self management, that her mortality was seriously endangered. These patients felt depreciated and inadequate, responding with overt anger or almost overwhelming periodic or continual depression or desire to withdraw not only from contact with offending individuals, but also from a hostile and punishing world.

The third category of work problems comprised a constellation of diverse *personal attitudes* brought by the respondent to the work setting, that often interacted with or gave rise to unpleasant conditions in the work environment. Among these were strong expectations that the patient would be met by attitudes such as she had evidenced towards others returning to the worksite after a bout with cancer. These anticipated reactions did not always materialize, to the patient's surprise, but her defensive apprehension sometimes led others to avoid her as "too touchy." There were also instances of deep uneasiness about how to counter solicitude or shunning, anxiety about how to demonstrate continued independence and productivity, anger at being stigmatized and singled out "by fate" for "punishment" for a nebulous *something*. While such attitudes also were noted among male respondents, the feelings of shame and guilt were more marked among women, as was cyclical or persistent depression. These personal attitudes were more prevalent among BC and WC women with mastectomies and YS patients with Hodgkin's Disease.

Some third-party interviews or patient descriptions of behavior suggested to the researchers the probability that the actions the woman described as "discrimination" or "unfair" had been precipitated by her own, or was a continuation of pre-cancer work behavior. Such instances were classified either as "workplace" or "personal" attitudes rather than "gross discrimination." Thus, interviews with five employers whom S.F. identified and consented to have contacted disclosed that she had lost four jobs because of personality conflicts prior to the cancer's detection and, before her mastectomy, already had been notified that her performance on Job Five was unsatisfactory. When R.T. was fired from the one-employee coffee-and-doughnut shop because she regaled customers with explicit gory details of her surgery despite their complaints and the owner's reiterated warnings, the dismissal was not classified as gross discrimination even though R.T. alleged the employer could not "stand to be around" someone with cancer she might "catch." Hence, the 25 percent of WC-reported instances of gross discrimination, 43 percent of the BC-reported situations, and the third of the YS-reported incidents of workplace discrimination should be construed as conservative estimates.

SOME COPING PATTERNS

The aggregated data from the three studies underscored not only the depth of the significant psychological and social—as well as economic—meanings of work to people in our society, but the compelling implications for the recovered cancer patient to establish and maintain an identity in the world of work as testimony to her continued value as an individual. This is tellingly illustrated in F.P.'s anguish when she said to the researcher, "I received two death sentences: one when the doctor told me I had cancer, and the other when my employer told me he could not keep me on because of the cancer even though I was able to do the work."

How did the patient-respondents reconcile their health and work requirements? Some simply did not disclose the diagnosis to anyone at work, confining time for diagnosis and treatment to non-work times. Some members of employee group health plans avoided claiming reimbursement if they thought (without necessarily knowing) management would learn of the cancer diagnosis through insurance reports. Several who could be designated as dependents in a spouse's employee health plan elected this option even though the spouse would have to pay for the dependent's coverage and the respondent's own employer already provided her with employee health benefits. Several mortgaged their homes or incurred other heavy debts for the immediate or long-term medical costs. Two reported that they represented themselves as medically indigent unemployed when the cancer was discovered, one going so far as to divorce her husband in order to qualify for public medical assistance, and the other not divulging her employment history to be sure that no revealing queries would be directed to the employer she expected to rehire her when her "leave" had ended. And several, especially WC clerks and lower-paid BC respondents, had to resort to public agencies for health and economic assistance.

The interviews disclosed that some employees characteristically were careful not to divulge personal health information either before or after the cancer diagnosis; their sense of personal privacy—and, sometimes, unwillingness to have women deemed "weak"—dictated such secrecy, although they did file claims for medical reimbursements. Information about health, including the cancer history, was withheld from employers more often by women than men. One possibility is that it was easier for them to do so because fewer women were in group health plans in their own workplaces; they were more often dependents in the husband's health plan and any report of medical reimbursement would not appear in her personnel record. Another is the belief of women respondents that cancer increased their vulnerability to sex-related job discrimination.

Yet more women than men were inclined to tell friends and associates at work (not superiors) about the cancer. In contrast, men generally were less reluctant to report the nature of the diagnosis but did not discuss with others either symptoms or any apprehension they might have felt about what these portended. But among male and female respondents in all the studies a clear pattern was evident that with each successive unsuccessful attempt to obtain or change jobs there was less and less inclination among job-seekers to mention the cancer in response to inquiries about health history. Indeed, a persistent and frequent query from study respondents and others to this writing is, "Should I tell about the cancer?"

Many of the women, especially in the BC group, accepted apathetically some of the overt and covert hostility and fear directed toward them. One respondent said, "This is just more 'punishment' as though the cancer isn't enough 'punishment'; what's the point of fighting?" But others mobilized the emotional and physical energy to retain control of the working phase of their lives even if to stem the progression of the disease might seem futile. This was more marked among the adults with supportive social systems—spouse, caring adult children or other relatives, close friends (often in the work situation). It also was sharply apparent among young respondents with close-knit parental ties and devoted siblings, some encouraging school personnel, and doctors the young patients described as treating them with respect and dignity. Also evident among the YS group was that motivation to persist in attaining educational and vocational goals was more sustained and effective when the caring parents were both employed and at least one had some college education.

On the job, patients availed themselves of opportunities to demonstrate continuing capability and worth as employees, to "prove" to the employer that the investment in the employee's training and retention over time was productive, not wasted. They assiduously avoided absences, even under circumstances that other employees would not hesitate over. Moreover, some patients volunteered for overtime tasks that could be construed as evidence of the patient's competence, unimpaired health, and loyal devotion to the job. Pervasive was the determination to demonstrate that the recovered cancer patient was not "handicapped" or "disabled". The noteworthy exception was among girls (and boys) with cancer of the bone or soft tissues who had experienced amputation. After repeated rejections for jobs because of cancer history, some wondered whether they might indeed be "disabled" even though good prostheses enabled them to perform the same tasks as others. Especially when the cancer preceded or occurred in the developmental stage characterized by apprehension about body image, such respondents tended toward severe depression that deepened as the search for work continued to be fruitless.

WORKING WOMEN AND CAREGIVING RESPONSIBILITIES

So far in this paper we have surveyed the work-related experiences and problems encountered by female former cancer patients. Their problems also "spill over" into the lives of their caregivers as well, who tend to be women (mothers, daughters, wives of male patients). The striking similarities in experiences make it worthwhile to summarize a small number of interviews with the caregivers themselves.

The employed caregivers interviewed about their experiences did indeed describe common pressures: conflicts between time and energy demands on the job and in the home; fears that anxieties about the patient and necessary absences in relation to them would lead to loss of a job needed for both economic and psychological reasons; difficulties within the family because values and expectations of filial piety toward an ill parent competed with the needs of spouse and children, or because concentration on the child with pediatric cancer diverted maternal attention from other children, or preoccupation with husband's cancer caused their working mother to neglect children.

The interviews with the caregiving working women reinforced the prevalent notion (Horowitz, 1985) that the primary responsibility for caring for elderly parents was assumed by daughters rather than by sons; even when the invalid was her spouse's parent, the working wife carried more nurturing responsibility, especially if the parent-in-law was in the family home. And when the parent lived elsewhere, travel costs and time often were added burdens.

Almost all of the caregiving women referred to periods of extreme exhaustion resulting from arduous continual tasks of moving, lifting, cleaning the patient—chores less likely among male family members, although they might share in feeding, medicating, cheering the patient. And all spoke of the strain of worry about the course and eventual outcome of the illness.

But certain elements in relation to the care of a cancer patient *were* different. A few caregivers spoke of being newly avoided by some coworkers (and friends outside the workplace) when it became known they were caring for a husband or parent in the home who had cancer. "They thought of me," said one, "as a kind of typhoid Mary!" Several described efforts to find better jobs, or jobs more accommodating to the caregiving needs (hours, location, etc.), but clinging to the same one because health benefits for a dependent with cancer would be denied elsewhere. More common, however, especially if the cancer patient was a child, was the continuing display of compassion toward the caregiver, and concrete and intangible offers of help both in personal and work situations—a sharp contrast to many of the experiences reported by cancer patients. The empathetic reactions provided an important support to some of the caregivers: they could channel some of their fears and pressures into responsive ears in the workplace, thereby gaining some emotional relief that freed them to continue coping with stresses at home. Some of these women wondered how they would have "survived" without the job and fellow workers to drain off some of the distress.

Attending a cancer patient differed from caregiving in other health situations in several ways. One was the frequency with which shame and guilt attached to this disease. For example, the C's, interviewed because of his rectal cancer, whispered throughout the BC interview that "no one knows, not even our son," and they were taking no chance that Mr. C's employer would learn of the cancer. Mrs. C tried to share and relieve Mr. C of some of his shame, but was consumed with self-guilt because she did not know how, except also to whisper. Bound to secrecy, and without any outlet for her feelings, she reported to the interviewer she expected to be fired (and was) because she could not concentrate on the technical work assigned her and could not tell anyone why.

Caregivers spoke of how hard it was to support and encourage the husband to cope with his illness and then help him deal with the hostility and fear he encountered on returning to work. Similarly, working mothers invested much effort in encouraging children with cancer to follow normal pursuits. For many, this also required constant vigilance about how others were behaving towards these children: teachers who treated them as "different," parents of other children who did not permit them to associate with the sick child because of the dread "cancer." One mother, a school employee, was threatened with dismissal because she challenged the gym teacher's exclusion of the child with an artificial leg, insisting to the teacher than even if Gerda fell, she had to learn to "pick herself up and go on; that will be her life." Another mother spent many days explaining to school personnel that her leukemic daughter should be allowed to associate freely with other children even if her hair had fallen out! Several mothers spoke of fears about children who were suicidal and did not understand that death would not reunite them with a sibling or grandparent who had died of cancer.

To help spouses and children cope with external relationships that were strained by the cancer not only consumed much emotional effort, but generally had to be handled during work hours and became a constant job threat for some of the women. And it appeared not unusual for some of the working mothers to wonder how much responsibility accrued to them for the fact that the child was ill; to fuel this conflict with guilt because they thought of the father's departure from the family following the diagnosis as an extension of "punishment" because of the child's cancer; and to be ambivalent about whether to abandon the job and devote full time to the patient's care even when her earnings were their primary or only means of support.

QUO VADEMUS?

The interviews with working women—caregivers or recovered patients—disclosed the vestigial impacts of ancient attitudes on contemporary life and work. Their burdens as patients or caregivers were grossly distorted by the heritage of metaphors and misinformation that shaped certain attitudes held by the patients themselves as well as by others in the workplace and profoundly influenced the quality of the individual's work and personal life. Given the importance of the work ethic in our society and the special meanings of work to the recovered cancer patients, whose numbers increase steadily, one must wonder how we can effectively proceed to change the idea that cancer is shameful, contagious, leprous?

One means is through legislation. For example, HR 1294, recently introduced by Congressman Mario Biaggi to protect the work-able cancer patient from actions and attitudes that adversely affect work status and opportunities, would provide a national vehicle to oppose workplace discrimination affecting persons with a cancer history. (Such legislation programs now exist only in California and Vermont).

But even were HR 1294 to become law and employers enjoined from discriminating against cancer patients, many women in the work force, affected by their own or another's cancer, would benefit only from a more personal kind of support system. The spreading movement of employee assistance programs and industrial social work services constitute one such system. This resource for personal counseling and staff training about cancer benefits employees and management, but has not yet been fully exploited. In the same vein, the growing movement of community support networks for care of the elderly or other special groups provides a model, if not actual service, for use by caregivers to cancer patients of various age groups and with their special problems relating to the nature of the disease and community and personal attitudes about it.

How to deal with attitudinal barriers in the work (and school) environment constitutes a challenge that affects many aspects of the cancer patient's life and expectations. Some insight into the nature of the challenge is to be found in this excerpt from a cancer patient's recent letter to the author:

> Where do I and other folks with cancer histories go for the courage to keep living? The diagnosis was frightening. Then my job as a dietitian was no longer there because my breast had been removed . . . My husband had trouble hiding feelings of revulsion . . . When the third place turned me down I began running around and screaming "What am I going to do? Where shall I go?" I calmed down and returned to the market place to shop again for a job. A job is more than my profession. It is my connection with life. Where shall I go?

Where, indeed?

REFERENCES

Feldman, F.L. (1976). *Work and Cancer Health Histories: A Study of Experiences of Recovered Patients*. San Francisco: American Cancer Society California Division, Inc.

Feldman, F.L. (1978). *Work and Cancer Health Histories: A Study of the Experiences of Recovered Blue-Collar Workers*. San Francisco: American Cancer Society California Division, Inc.

Feldman, F.L. (1980). *Work and Cancer Health Histories: Work Expectations and Experiences of Youth (Ages 13–23) with Cancer Histories*. San Francisco: American Cancer Society California Division, Inc.

Horowitz, A. (1985). Sons and daughters as caregivers to older parents: Differences in role performance and consequences. *Gerontologist* 25(6): 612–618.
McKenna, R. (1973). Analysis of Case Histories: Employability Problems of the Recovered Cancer Patient. Report of ad hoc committee. San Francisco: American Cancer Society California Divison, Inc.
Stone, R.W. (1975). Employing the recovered cancer patient. Cancer 36:285–286.
Wheatley, G.M., Cunnick, W.R. et al. (1972). *The Employment of Persons with a History of Treatment for Cancer*. New York: Metropolitan Life Insurance Company.

Women and Hospice Care

Jana Hach, MSW, ACSW
Sarah A. Wilson, RN, MS

ABSTRACT. The hospice movement has grown extensively in the last ten years. This article examines the role of women in hospice, components of hospice care and a profile of 544 admissions to an inpatient hospice unit over a five year period. Case studies are given to illustrate the needs of women in hospice. Regulatory processes facing hospice programs today are reviewed.

Hospice is a concept of care, not a specific facility or agency. While its origins can be traced to ancient times, today it represents a rapidly growing system of care for the terminally ill. Its primary goals are "to control pain, ensure general comfort (both spiritual and mental), assure a dignified death for the patient, and give support and comfort to his family" (Leone, 1982).

The hospice concept is of particular interest in the context of women and cancer. About 90% of hospice patients have a diagnosis of cancer (Greer and Mor, 1986). Since women now account for just under half of all cancer deaths in the United States (Silverberg and Lubera, 1986), they comprise a large proportion of the people receiving hospice care. In fact, slightly over half of the hospice patients studied in the National Hospice Survey were women (Greer et al., 1986). The coordination and management of the patient's everyday care is almost always in the hands of a female nurse (Greene, 1984). In addition, women have played a major role in the founding and development of hospice.

Jana Hach, formerly Administrative Director of Mount Sinai Hospice, is a psychotherapist with Mount Sinai Medical Center, Milwaukee, WI 53208. Sarah A. Wilson is Assistant Professor of Nursing at Marquette University, Milwaukee, WI 53233.

HISTORICAL OVERVIEW

The French word "hospice" is derived from the Latin "hospes" which means a place where a guest was received, but the modern medical usage of the term began in Britain in the last century. The Irish Sisters of Charity, inspired by the work of Sister Mary Aikenhead (a co-worker of Florence Nightingale), opened a hospice near Dublin in 1879 (McNulty and Holderby, 1983). Sister Aikenhead considered death to be a beginning of a final journey, and had called her nursing home by the name of a resting place on a medieval pilgrimage to the Holy Land (Cohen, 1978).

By the end of the nineteenth century, there were numerous hospices in England. The hospice most like the one in Dublin was St. Joseph's Hospice, founded by the English Sisters of Charity in 1906. It was there that in the 1950s and 1960s Cicely Saunders did research in the control of pain. St. Christopher's in London, which she founded in 1967, became a model for present day hospices.

In 1971, Hospice, Inc. was formed in New Haven, Connecticut as the first facility of its kind in the United States (Goldenberg, 1979), and drew heavily on the English experience. Since then the number of programs has undergone explosive growth. In 1978 the U.S. General Accounting Office reported 59 existing hospices with 73 in planning stages (Buckingham, 1982, p. 455). There were more than 800 at the time of the first JCAH hospice survey in 1981, and an update in 1983–84 counted 1,429 (Cunningham, 1985). The National Hospice Association lists 700 provider member hospice programs as of November, 1985.

LEGITIMIZATION OF HOSPICE AND DEVELOPMENT OF STANDARDS

Considering the short time since the hospice movement began in America, it is remarkable how quickly guidelines and even formal standards have developed. During 1981–3, the Joint Commission on Accreditation of Hospitals (JCAH) conducted a study of numbers and characteristics of hospice providers, funded by the W. K. Kellogg Foundation of Battle Creek, Michigan. The results, published by the Commission (JCAH, 1981; McCann, 1985) gave rise to development of hospice standards and, in 1984, establishment of the JCAH Accreditation Program for Hospice Care.

The accreditation process became mandatory in 1985 for any hospital based hospice unit located in a hospital which was undergoing the JCAH survey on the rest of the facility. As of October 1, 1985, 50 hospice programs nationally were JCAH Accredited with 35 more scheduled to be surveyed.

The following are some highlights of the standards (JCAH, 1983):

- designation of the patient and his family or some other primary careperson as the unit of care.
- establishment of an interdisciplinary team, including at least physician, nursing services, psychological/social work services, and spiritual and bereavement services.
- continuity of care between hospital and home setting.
- availability 24 hours a day.

Further impetus for development of standards was the Tax Equity and Fiscal Responsibility Act of 1982, which provided a Medicare home hospice service benefit. Final Medicare Hospice Benefit regulations under this act were published in the Federal Register on December 16, 1985. This law introduced a voluntary certification procedure.

As of October 1, 1985, 205 hospice programs were Medicare Certified. The breakdown in settings of these programs is:

- 98 Home Health Agency Based
- 45 Hospital Based
- 10 Skilled Nursing Facility
- 52 Freestanding

This benefit requires that 80% of the care be delivered in the patient's home. This home care focus combined with the DRG factor in hospitals limiting the length of stay of hospice patients is causing a dramatic shift in hospice care towards the home care market.

As illustrated by the breakdown of the Medicare Certified hospice programs, hospice care crosses many other types of licensed health care. More than 20 states are working with hospice licensure on the state level to set minimum standards for hospice programs.

The direction of hospice programming in the future will be cost conscious, delivered at least 80% in the home setting, and will continue to be primarily developed by and implemented by women. It is to the credit of the hospice movement that it has persisted and flourished in an era of health care cutbacks. Although regulatory processes will change the format of some of the smaller programs, these processes also insure that hospice has a role in health care for decades to come.

RESEARCH ON HOSPICE SYSTEMS

The extraordinary growth of this movement in the past decade has given rise to a burgeoning literature. The July/August 1984 issue of the American Cancer Society's journal CA contained five feature articles on hospice care, and Haworth Press (publisher of this journal) introduced Vol 1, No. 1 of the Hospice Journal in Spring, 1985. Other journals have also published special issues on hospice care, such as the Vol. 2, Nos. 1–2 of the quarterly journal Death Education, and the March, 1979 issue of Hospital Progress.

Nevertheless, or perhaps because of the newness of the field, little quantitative data is available on the characteristics of either hospices themselves or their patients. Many early studies were done very informally, and much of the recent literature is descriptive or philosophical.

In 1980, the Robert Wood Johnson Foundation and the John A. Hartford Foundation cosponsored (with the Health Care Financing Administration) the National Hospice Study. The findings of this three-year study of 1754 hospice and nonhospice patients in 26 hospices and 14 conventional oncologic institutions were published in a special issue of the Journal of Chronic Diseases (vol. 39, no. 1, 1986). Using a "quasi-experimental" design, Greer et al. (1986) reported that half of all patients died within 35 days of admission, that nearly 20% stayed 10 days or less, that 90% had diagnoses of cancer, and that over 90% have an involved caretaker, usually a member of the family. Compared with terminal cancer patients in conventional care facilities, hospice patients were significantly less likely to receive chemotherapy, surgery, radiation, or diagnostic tests. They were more likely to receive social services. Their quality of life was no worse than that of conventional patients.

In the remainder of this paper, we describe several cases which demonstrate the "non-typical" nature of hospice patients, followed by a survey of the patient makeup of one institution.

CASE DESCRIPTIONS

Everyone has his own perception of who a hospice patient might be. Many think of any elderly parent or grandparent who has the family unit available to assist them with their needs. The following case descriptions of three women serviced at an inpatient hospice in Milwaukee, Wisconsin illustrate that the hospice patient can be any age and does not necessarily have a primary care person available to them. In such cases, the hospice team becomes a surrogate extended family.

Jane is a 21 year old retarded woman with leukemia whose parents have been her primary caretakers. She has utilized the inpatient hospice unit on three occasions before her death. She would be admitted during crisis times when her platelets dropped to 20,000. She has been transfused for comfort reasons. Although her parents share the caregiving responsibilities, the father's employment gives him an outlet. The mother spends the night at hospice seeing the patient through bad dreams and worried nights. Like many facing death, Jane is afraid of the dark and being alone. During the three months in the hospice program, the family was followed at home by frequent telephone contacts as they wanted to provide the hands-on care themselves. The patient's mother was encouraged to seek more outside interests, as centering her life around the one adopted daughter would present a high risk during bereavement. At hospice, Jane's poodle was a daily visitor and even positively influenced the morale of other visiting families. Many staff members attended Jane's wake. To be able to receive hospital care in a homelike environment was reassuring to this stressed family. The team which had a ratio of one nurse to every three patients, had the time and energy to decrease anxiety and manage symptoms to provide care for this family system.

Chris is a 44 year old single parent with twin 16 year old daughters. Other than siblings, she did not have a primary care person available to her. Pain management requiring high doses of morphine sulfate was the primary focus on admission. Once Chris's pain was under control, the morphine was decreased and valuable interaction with her children became possible. She had not spoken to her daughters about her death. The girls were aware of a limited prognosis but had not discussed this with anyone. The daughters would visit, ask about pain, then stay quietly at the bedside reading. A family conference with nursing, social services, the physician, the patient and her daughters broke the ice about discussing her death and also allowed planning as to who would raise these children. New openness enabled these daughters to become involved in caring for their mother in such ways as assisting with washing her face and making her comfortable before they left at night. This experience has given a brief but meaningful time of interaction where these children can touch and receive from their mother.

When Chris died, her daughters were present and were comfortable crying with and being held by the hospice staff. They face many changes in their young lives including a move to another city, changing schools and adjusting to life with a different parent; however this time at hospice made the experience of their mother's death a little more human, a little more open and slightly more bearable.

Lile is an 82 year old woman who broke her hip at home, dragged herself to a commode and sat there for three days until she was discovered and admitted with metastatic cancer, a large sacral decubitus and the broken bone. She was depressed and her pain was out of control. Controlling the pain, use of a mood elevator and specialty bed with an air flotation system all enabled this woman to die after having some quality time. She had been a recluse; even her minister admitted he was reluctant to visit her. After intervention by the hospice team, she enjoyed conversations with volunteers, laughed at times and died with the hospice team really being her primary care persons. She was afraid of thunder and when there was a storm she would receive calls from volunteers offering to come and sit with her.

STATISTICAL PROFILE OF ONE HOSPICE

Mount Sinai Hospice is a ten bed inpatient hospice unit which is part of Mount Sinai Medical Center in Milwaukee, Wisconsin. All of the inpatient hospice admissions for a five year period were tallied to determine the age, sex and primary diagnoses of those patients served.

Of the 544 inpatient admissions, 48% were men and 52% were women. The mean age of the male patients was 67.4 years compared to 64.9 for women. This is reflected in Table 1. The majority of the young women served had cancer of the uterus or ovary, were single parents, and did not have a primary care person available to them at home. This, combined with the acute nature of the care needed at the end of their lives, makes them a patient

Table 1

Number of Inpatient Admissions
By Age and Sex
Mount Sinai Hospice, Milwaukee, WI
1981 to 1986

Age	Male		Female	
	No.	(%)	No.	(%)
20-24			4	(1.4%)
25-29			6	(2.1%)
30-34	2	(0.8%)	6	(2.1%)
35-39	2	(0.8%)	5	(1.8%)
40-44	7	(2.7%)	8	(2.9%)
45-49	15	(5.7%)	11	(3.9%)
50-54	17	(6.5%)	28	(9.9%)
55-59	35	(13.3%)	22	(7.8%)
60-64	19	(7.2%)	39	(13.8%)
65-69	43	(16.4%)	39	(13.8%)
70-74	47	(17.9%)	42	(15.0%)
75-79	32	(12.2%)	41	(14.5%)
80-84	30	(11.5%)	20	(7.1%)
85-89	10	(3.8%)	9	(3.2%)
90-94	2	(0.8%)	2	(0.7%)
95+	1	(0.4%)		
TOTAL	262	(100.0%)	282	(100.0%)

population probably not seen in home hospice. Men are often cared for by their wives or families except in the elderly population where the wife may have health problems of her own. This may explain why fewer men than women are served in our inpatient hospice setting, and why they tend to be older. However, women have been found to have more positive attitudes towards hospice as they have toward health services in general and therefore may use all health services more than men do (Rainey, 1985).

Table 2 shows the breakdown of the diagnoses of patients over the five year period. Of the 262 men admitted, 95% had a primary

Table 2

Primary Diagnosis of 544 Hospice Inpatient Admissions, By Sex, 1981 to 1986

	Males		Females	
Diagnosis	No.	(%)	No.	(%)
CANCER	249	(95.0%)	257	(91.1%)
Oral cavity	17	(6.5%)	6	(2.1%)
Stomach	10	(3.8%)	2	(0.7%)
Colon, rectum	33	(12.6%)	37	(13.1%)
Pancreas	6	(2.3%)	13	(4.6%)
Lung	89	(34.0%)	52	(18.4%)
Melanoma	7	(2.7%)	2	(0.7%)
Breast	0		49	(17.4%)
Uterine	0		18	(6.4%)
Ovary	0		17	(6.0%)
Vulvar, vaginal	0		8	(2.8%)
Prostate	22	(8.4%)	0	
Urinary tract	17	(6.5%)	5	(1.8%)
Brain	17	(6.5%)	16	(5.7%)
Lymphoma, leukemia	10	(3.8%)	10	(3.5%)
Multiple myeloma	3	(1.1%)	4	(1.4%)
Other	18	(6.9%)	18	(6.4%)
Chronic Obstructive Pulmonary Disease	6	(2.3%)	3	(1.1%)
AIDS	3	(1.1%)	0	
Cardiac disease	1	(0.4%)	5	(1.8%)
Renal failure	1	(0.4%)	1	(0.4%)
ALS	1	(0.4%)	2	(0.7%)
Other	1	(0.4%)	14	(5.0%)
TOTAL	262	(100.0%)	282	(100.0%)

diagnosis of cancer, while 91% of the 282 women had a cancer diagnosis. There will probably be an increase in noncancer male patients as the AIDS patients in the Milwaukee area require terminal care.

The distribution of cancer diagnoses of the hospice patients served at Mount Sinai Hospice closely follows that of estimated cancer deaths of site and sex nationally (American Cancer Society, 1985). The major difference is a much lower percentage of leukemia patients seen in hospice. The leukemia patient is often treated in a traditional setting because of the blood transfusions and frequent laboratory tests. The leukemia patient also tends to be younger and can be cared for in the home setting by a primary care person.

Many argue the merits of inpatient versus home hospice care. The reality is that both options need to be available to patients and families, with a strong interface between these parts of the hospice program. The continuity of care required by JCAH standards benefits the patient and family.

REFERENCES

American Cancer Society. (1985). Facts and Figures, 1985. New York, NY: ACS.

Buckingham, R.W., & Lupu, D. (1982). A comparative study of hospice services in the United States. *Am J Public Health* 72:455–463.

Cohen, K. (1979). Hospice Prescription for Terminal Care. Rockville, MD: Aspen Systems Corp.

Cunningham, R.M. (1985, April 16) The evolution of hospice. *Hospitals*. pp. 124–126.

Goldenberg, L.S. (1979, April) Hospice: To humanize dying. *Bull Am Coll Surg* 64(4): 6–9.

Green, P.E. (1984). The pivotal role of the nurse in hospice care. *CA-A Cancer Journal for Clinicians* 34:204–205.

Greer, D.S., & Mor, V. (1986) An overview of National Hospice Study findings. *J Chron Dis* 39:5–7.

Greer, D.S., Mor. V., Morris, J.N., Sherwood, S., Kidder, D., & Birnbaum, H. (1986). An alternative in terminal care: results of the National Hospice Study. *J Chron Dis* 39:9–26.

Joint Commission on Accreditation of Hospitals. (1981). JCAH Hospice Project Interim Report, Phase 1. Chicago, IL: JCAH.

Joint Commission on Accreditation of Hospitals. (1983). Hospice Standards Manual. Chicago, IL: JCAH.

Leone, L.A. (1982) The concept of hospice. *CA-A Cancer Journal for Clinicians* 32:141–143.

McCann, B.A. (1985). The Hospice Project Report. Chicago, IL: JCAH.

McNulty, E.G., & Holderby, R.A. (1983). Hospice: A Caring Challenge. Springfield, IL: Charles C. Thomas.

Rainey, L.C., Crane, L., Breslow, D.V., & Ganz, P. (1984). Cancer patients' attitudes towards hospice services. *CA-A Cancer Journal for Clinicians* 34:191–201.

Silverberg, E., & Lubera, J. (1986). Cancer statistics, 1986. *CA-A Cancer Journal for Clinicians* 36:9–25.

The Deadliest Delusion: Unproven Methods in the Management of Cancer

Helene G. Brown

ABSTRACT. In spite of major advances in cancer treatment over the past decades, unproven or ineffective methods of treatment continue to be offered to the public by unqualified or unscrupulous practitioners. These methods fall into five categories: devices, tests, drugs, diets, and psychological methods, as well as combinations of these. The emotional, physical, and financial burdens of cancer treatment make cancer patients and their families especially vulnerable to the pitch of these operators. Participation in worthless treatments can lead to loss of life or prolongation of illness which might otherwise have been avoided through orthodox cancer treatment. Ineffective treatments can generally be recognized by application of some simple guidelines. Lack of faith in the medical care system is an important motivation in the choice of alternative therapies. Health practitioners have an obligation to be sensitive to patients' needs, and to provide emotional as well as medical support, to communicate openly with patients and families, and to nurture the trust that will prevent abandonment of traditional medical care in favor of quackery.

Great strides are being made in cancer therapy. As other papers in this volume have documented (Devesa, 1986; Funch, 1986), the mortality rates from some cancers have fallen and survival rates increased during the past few decades. Cancer found before it spreads is often curable. Even after some metastasis has taken place, quality of life, long term survival, and in many cases cure, can be achieved through the use of surgery, radiation, chemotherapy, immuno-therapy, hormonal therapy and combinations of these.

Nevertheless, cancer continues to be the second leading cause of

Helene G. Brown is Vice-President, American Cancer Society, and Co-Director, Divison of Cancer Control, Jonsson Comprehensive Cancer Center at UCLA, 10920 Wilshire Boulevard #1106, Los Angeles, CA 90024.

death in the United States. Not all cancer patients are cured, and treatment and its aftermath is not always easy or comfortable (see other papers in this volume: Penman et al., 1986; Ulbricht, 1986). When cancer treatment is required, patients and their families must make judgments from a base of knowledge, understanding, and reason, and not by emotion. Yet, in many cases, even among the most knowledgeable, emotions will play a major role in the judgment process. It is this inevitable intense emotional involvement by the patient, the family and friends that cause them to be exploited by those selling, promoting or administering unproven remedies.

Women, in particular, shoulder major responsibility in avoiding the seduction of worthless approaches and false promises which so often lead to deadly delusion, because of the long recognized role that they play as the "health educators" in the family as well as in the community at large. It is therefore critically important that women know and recognize not only what is good in matters of cancer management but what is not good as well, which for the purposes of this paper, will be "quackery" in cancer, or the use of unproven methods.

Medical quackery remains a persistent problem in the United States, but it is not a modern phenomenon. Throughout written history, useless salves, escharotics (substances which produce a scab) for external lesions, teas, poultices made from cobwebs and arsenic, diets, urine derivatives of both man and beast, machines and devices, vitamins and exotic formulas of all sorts have been proposed as worthwhile approaches for the prevention, detection and cure of cancer (American Cancer Society, 1982).

The modern purveyor of worthless methods is not as easy to recognize as the snake-oil salesman of days past. The modern charlatan often uses sophisticated medical terminology and may actually refer to publications which can best be termed pseudoscience (Barrett, 1980). Especially alarming is the fact that purveyors of unorthodox therapies can be physicians themselves. A University of Pennsylvania survey found that 60% of "unorthodox practitioners" were M.D.'s, and that the therapies offered usually combined conventional with alternative methods (Cassileth, et al., 1984).

The use of unproven methods, whether by misguided doctors or outright peddlers of fraud, leads to the exploitation of patients, the depletion of their savings and the loss of life or of extended well-being among those who could have been successfully treated using recognized regimens.

TYPES OF UNPROVEN METHODS

The American Cancer Society has categorized, documented, and published materials on more than seventy individual methods. Table 1 shows a sample of some of them. Most fall into five categories: (1) devices, (2) tests, (3) drugs, (4) diets, and (5) psychological approaches, as well as combinations of these.

Devices

A variety of devices have in the past been promoted as cures for cancer, although devices have lost some of their popularity in recent years. Most devices tend to be similar, equipped with impressive looking dials and lights on the front or top. They come in a variety of sizes ranging from ones as small as a candy box to others as large as a console floor model. Commonly, a wire, which is inserted via a jack into the box, has a plate or pad on the opposite end. The pad

TABLE 1

Partial list of statements on

Unproven Methods of Cancer Management

prepared by the American Cancer Society

Anti-Cancer Factor in Clams (Mercenene)	Hoxsey Method or Hoxsey Chemotherapy
Anticancergen Z-50 and Zuccala Lytic Test	Immuno Augmentive Therapy (IAT)
Antineol	Iscador
Bamfolin	Kanfer Neuromuscular or Handwriting Test
Bio-Medical Detoxification Therapy	KC-555
Bonifacio Anticancer Goat Serum	Koch Antitoxins
Carcin and Neo-carcin	Krebiozen and Carcalon
Carzodelan	Laetrile
Chaparral Tea	Livingston Vaccine
Diamond Carbon Compound	Mucorhicin
Dimethyl Sulfoxide (DMSO)	Multiple Enzyme Therapy
Electronic Devices	Orgone Energy Devices
Fresh Cell Therapy	Polonine
Gerson Method	Spears Hygienic System
Grape Diet	Ultraviolet Blood Irradiation Intravenous Treatment
H-11	Zen Macrobiotic Diet

is placed on the body where the lesion is said to exist, the dials are set according to instructions, and the plug is inserted into an electrical outlet. On occasion dials and meters on the box react, indicating activity.

"Treatment" is thus delivered in the patient's own home. At-home treatment may increase the attractiveness of the method for some patients. Many people enjoy the thought of participating in their own treatment regimen by applying the treatment themselves. Not traveling to the physician's office or hospital is also an attractive feature. For some, merely viewing the moving meter needle may be gratifying, or may make the patient feel that "something is being done." Devices have a magic lantern effect, even though they usually contain only an electrical circuit responsible for moving the lights and dials.

One typical device was described as follows:

> The Electron-O-Ray Models were suitcase-type units. They contained a combination of electronic circuits with a control panel containing pilot lights, switches, and a series of dials intended for use in determining the identity of diseased organs. A "detector plate" purported to locate the point of maximum reaction and thus determine the location of the disease in the body. They also had a "food test plate" which could select a diet for the patient. (American Cancer Society, 1965).

Tests

Simple, effective screening tests which will reveal the presence of any cancer in an asymptomatic individual before it spreads are, of course, a major goal of researchers and the public health community. The utility of such tests is obvious since cancer detected at an early stage is curable in some sites and leads to extended survival in many others. Thus the appeal of such a test is easy to understand. To date, however, there are no known universal detection methods for cancer. One test, the cervical Pap smear, is highly effective in the early detection and cure of cervical carcinoma. Mammography is in widespread use for detection of breast cancer.

The existence of such highly effective screening methods may enhance the credibility of quacks' claims for their methodologies. Because many people are already familiar with these legitimate tests, phony claims for a more comprehensive test are more easily believed.

They are sometimes promoted as a "pap test" for "cancer any place in the body" using urine, blood, skin, and even handwriting. Examples of unproven diagnostic tests for cancer are: Livingston Mycobacteria Test, Anthrone Color Test, Kelly Malignancy Test, and Urinary Chorionic Gonadotrophin Test (National Council Against Health Fraud, 1984).

It is not only the cancer patient who is the victim of unproven diagnostic and early detection tests. Fraudulent tests are used by the "worried well" as well, or by those who may have some condition other than cancer. The user of unproven diagnostic techniques may then be lured into the use of unproven treatments as well if the "test" is found to be positive and the patient led to believe that he or she has cancer. Such therapy is, of course usually curative precisely because the patient has never had cancer. Word of the "miracle cure" will be spread throughout the now-cured "victim's" social community, possibly entrapping other gullible people.

Drugs

Each decade seems to bring its own "miracle drug" for cancer, touted in the media and promoted politically. One of the biggest health furors of the 1950s was caused by the Hoxsey Herbal Tonic Treatment. In the 1960s, thousands of cancer patients eagerly sought that decade's cancer hope, krebiozen. Eventually, both of these were exposed as completely ineffective (Subcommittee on Unorthodox Therapies, 1983).

The 1970s brough Laetrile, also called Amygdalin and Vitamin B-17. The Food and Drug Administration has repeatedly refused to permit its use as a medicine, and obtained injunctions against its interstate shipment as a "vitamin" (Food and Drug Administration, 1977; Consumer Reports, 1977). Nevertheless, in response to public pressure, as many as 27 states have legalized its use. Recognizing this pressure, and seeing an obligation to respond to a major public health problem, a formal clinical trial of Laetrile was undertaken by the National Cancer Institute. The results, published in the New England Journal of Medicine in 1982, demonstrated conclusively that "Amygdalin (Laetrile) is a toxic drug that is not effective as a cancer treatment" (Moertel et al., 1982).

Despite this official condemnation, Laetrile continues to thrive in many so-called "cancer clinics" as an emotional and political success even while a scientific failure. Its promoters state that one must be a "trained metabolic physician" to get results with Laetrile. What this really means is that the drug will "work" only for Laetrile proponents and "working" does not necessarily meaning "curing." [To counter this assertion, the NCI clinical trial included a metabolic diet component along with Laetrile therapy. Even then, only the drug's proponents failed to be convinced of its worthlessness.]

Now, in the 1980s, we find Immuno Augmentative Therapy (IAT), DMSO, and various vaccine approaches aligning themselves with legitimate areas of research and technological advance. The promoters of IAT declined an offer by the National Cancer Institute for a collaborative evaluation of their method. Since they would reveal "neither the composition of the treatment materials nor the method of preparing them," an impartial scientific test has so far been impossible (American Cancer Society, 1984). Nevertheless, support groups made up of patients, families and friends, expound on the benefits of the therapy and are emotionally driven to "pass the good word" and lure patients from recognized, potentially beneficial treatment.

Diets

The importance of good nutrition and the relevance of a balanced diet to health are undisputed. Scientifically established relationships between diet and disease, including cancer and heart disease, exist. Some scientists believe that up to 70% of the cancers are dietary in origin (Doll and Peto, 1981). Adequate nutrition is especially important to the cancer patient both during and after treatment, to build resistance to infections and gain strength to recover normal function. Cancer therapy sometimes causes loss of appetite. Many medical practitioners may not be aware of the latest information on diet and disease or may not have the skill or interest to advise patients on the nutritional aspects of their disease. These factors may enhance the attractiveness and credibility of questionable dietary regimes, even for the patient who has already undergone a standard therapy.

Unproven nutritional methods are known by a variety of names such as "nutritional therapy," "metabolic therapy," "holistic therapy," "alternative therapy," and "non-toxic therapy." Each of these phrases strikes a responsive chord because of its dictionary meaning, but the actual regimens are at best not known to be useful and at worst may be nutritionally and metabolically destructive rather than helpful (Herbert, 1984). One example of a bizarre dietary regimen . . .

> . . . begins with an eight-ounce glass of juice each hour, a total of about 13 glasses a day. Included are carrot, apple, orange and "green" juices, the latter made from a mixture of vegetables, and three glasses daily of juice extracted from pressed raw liver. Patients also receive tablespoons of linseed oil, acidophilus-pepsin capsules, potassium solution, Lugol's solution (an iodine/potassium iodide solution) added to the juice, thyroid tablets, 300 mg of niacin daily, pancreatic enzymes, royal jelly capsules, and injections of vitamin B-12 mixed with liver. Except for the liver juice, the first four weeks' diet contains no protein from animal sources and is strictly vegetarian. (Lowell, 1986)

Unorthodox dietary "therapy" is quite common among cancer patients, even those undergoing standard treatment. Cassileth and associates found that 37% of patients undergoing both conventional and unorthodox treatments were receiving some form of unorthodox dietary regime, compared with 26% of those undergoing unorthodox treatment only (Cassileth et al., 1984).

Psychological Approaches

The psychological approaches to treatment of cancer are often based on the proposition that "stress" is a cause of cancer. Some psychological methods attempt to use "stress" reduction and other purported psychologically beneficial techniques as a cure for cancer. Imaging techniques (in which the patient attempts to "visualize" or imagine destruction of cancer cells), hypnosis, patient counseling without concurrent medical oversight, have all been used to "treat" cancer patients.

The main problem with questionable psychological approaches to cure cancer, or the use of interventions known to be helpful in stress reduction without a concurrent medical regime, is that the patient can be deprived of optimum medical care offering possibility of cure, increased survival time or palliation of physical symptoms associated with the disease.

On the face of it, stress management has great appeal as an adjunctive factor in treating cancer. Stress is an established or suspected factor in the causation and course of many diseases, including coronary heart disease, hypertension, diabetes, and other ailments. However, it has not been established, nor is it likely, that stress reduction will lead to the halting of the metastasis of an untreated malignancy or reduction in tumor mass. Yet in this area of unproven methodologies, the unwarranted logical leap is made. If one knows or suspects the cause of the disease, then its elimination will likely lead to a cure. A graphic counter-example to this reasoning is cigarette smoking. While it is certain that eliminating the use of tobacco will prevent the majority of future lung cancers from occurring, the elimination of use of tobacco after disease onset cannot lead to the cure of a lung lesion already manifest.

Stress reduction can be beneficial to a cancer patient in tolerating difficult treatment regimens and in managing the psychological burden of cancer. Such psycho-social interventions can be advantageous in aiding families of patients, often by providing a welcome adjunct to treatment, which enables them to exercise some control and actively participate in the management of the illness. Art as therapy, dance as therapy, stress reduction, laughter as medicine, psychological counseling and other valid adjuncts to treatment offered to cancer patients have their place, but their limitations must be recognized and accepted. Such benefits may even lead to prolongation of well-being for the patient. However, the claim that any of these alone will lead to cure has not been proven valid.

FACTORS CONTRIBUTING TO THE USE OF UNPROVEN METHODS

It is valuable to try to understand the many factors contributing to the sale and acceptance of unproven methods. These are just a few of the many reasons stated and unstated:

Cancer is among the complex, difficult illnesses (cancer, stroke, multiple sclerosis) which are the major killers in modern industrial societies. Since many of the less complex diseases have now been prevented or are totally curable, there is an expectation of cure for cancer as well.

Patients receiving alternative therapies often believe: (1) disease is caused by poor nutrition, or (2) disease is caused by worry or stress, and (3) that chemotherapy and radiation therapy are more harmful than helpful (Cassileth et al., 1984). This meshes well with the main messages of unproven therapies which hold that: (1) cancer is less a disease entity than a symptom of underlying toxicity or dysfunction, (2) remedies for these underlying dysfunctions are pleasant and do not have to include side effects, (3) therapy should be based in the home rather than the hospital, and (4) simple explanations can be given for cancer, such as "emotional stress" or "poor diet."

Cancer treatment is costly monetarily, emotionally and physically, but is not always effective. It is reasonable for the cancer victim or his or her family to want to seek another avenue. One way of counteracting this might be to present as realistically positive a picture as is warranted. Many patients have a sense that cancer is always fatal. They are unaware that survival from many cancers is common, that overall 50% of cancer is curable today, and that in some instances, like early, localized breast cancer, survival is 80% or better. Even when hope for cure must be abandoned, it should be emphasized that good medical and psycho-social care can extend life and provide a better death (see paper on hospice care elsewhere in this volume: Hach and Wilson, 1986).

Unproven methods are often said to have few or no side effects, in contrast to the admittedly harsh and toxic side effects sometimes produced by conventional chemotherapy. This is especially unfortunate since there has been significant progress in the treatment of cancer with drug therapy in the past decade or more, particularly in adjustment of dosages and reduction of side effects and toxicity.

After unsuccessful or partially successful treatment, when expectations are not fulfilled, a patient may turn to the practitioner who reports success using a kernel of truth upon which exaggerated claims are made or who fools the public with a sin of omission. He may describe a previous patient as "thriving" under a therapy when in reality that patient is found to be dead shortly after a report of "successful" treatment (Monaco, 1982).

The pressures from family and friends to "try harder and everything" is often more than a patient can endure. They are dependent on their family and friend network for support. Disagreement is distasteful and so it becomes easier to "switch" than to "fight," especially when orthodox medical treatments are lengthy and harsh.

Distrust of those in power and of the medical profession is widespread. Claims that there is a "medical trust" which will not permit a cancer cure to be brought to market has credibility among many patients and their families.

The media has created a more knowledgeable and questioning public. Advances in cancer research are published for the benefit of sharing information and encouraging further research. This exposure has increased the expectations of the public, who look eagerly to the daily newspapers and magazines for their source of new information. The lay public cannot automatically be expected to distinguish reports of legitimate research from those out of the mainstream.

RECOGNIZING UNPROVEN OR "QUACK" METHODS

Given the practically limitless variety and number of unproven methods, how can one distinguish such an offering from authentic treatment? Ten ways in which ineffective treatments can be recognized have been presented by the Subcommittee on Unorthodox Therapies of the American Society of Clinical Oncology (Subcommittee on Unorthodox Therapies, 1983).

1. Is the treatment based on an unproven theory?
2. Is there a purported need for special nutritional support?
3. Is there a claim for painless, nontoxic treatment?
4. Are claims published only in the mass media, and not in reputable "peer review" scientific journals?
5. Are claims for benefit merely compatible with a placebo effect?
6. Are the major promoters recognized experts in cancer treatment?
7. Do proponents claim benefit for use with proven methods of cancer treatment? for prolongation of life? for use as a cancer preventive?

8. Is there a claim that only specially trained physicians can produce results with their drug, or is the preparation a secret?
9. Do the promoters attack the medical and scientific "establishment"?
10. Is there a demand by promoters for "freedom of choice" regarding drugs?

In nearly every case of unproven methods examined by the ASCO Subcommittee, the answer to each of the above questions was "Yes," except for number 6, which was "No." Application of these simple guidelines can help to distinguish unproven methods from conventional medical practice quickly.

The ASCO has also suggested specific ways in which practitioners themselves can assist their patients in evaluating therapies based upon these 10 questions. One is to use reputable sources of information. Those who have access to computerized literature searches through their library or the NCI Cancer Information Service might commission a "search" of the literature on the therapy in question.

Libraries and computer data bases also contain professional directories which can be consulted in order to assess credentials of promoters of alternative therapies. Some of these include the *Directory of Medical Specialists*, and the directories of the American Federation of Clinical Oncologic Societies, the American Association for Cancer Research, and the American Society of Clinical Oncology. These directories list individuals who have recognition, special training and experience in the fields of cancer research and treatment. While excellent adjunctive counseling, nutritional advice, and social work are available through many agencies and resources, cancer itself remains a medical problem that must be dealt with through qualified medical personnel.

The patient should be warned about the "media" and its sometimes ill-advised promotion of "miracle" cures, devices and regimens. Even an intelligent, informed cancer patient who might otherwise see through these may be in a vulnerable state. Frank and open discussion by the physician, nurse, or other health professional will help the patient retain perspective.

The claim that the scientific, medical, government and pharmaceutical "establishment" are in a "conspiracy" to prevent a cancer cure should be discussed. One reason often stated by the promoters of unproven methods is that treating cancer is so lucrative. (The ASCO Committee points out that these promoters rarely mention the amount of money they derive from their patients.) Frank and open discussion with the patient will help provide perspective on this issue. The controlled clinical trials that have taken place with drugs like Laetrile should be cited in such a discussion.

The tenth ASCO rule merits special discussion. Numerous promoters have raised the argument that the public's freedom of choice would be limited if they were not permitted to promote and sell their products. The freedom-of-choice argument is a linchpin of nearly all attempts to gain legitimacy, and has proved especially useful in convincing state legislators to legalize various methods. Use of this argument is faulty and may pose difficult legal and ethical dilemmas and issues (see also the paper on ethics in cancer studies elsewhere in this volume: Soskolne, 1986).

In fact, American law has been quite clear on this point for over three-quarters of a century. Beginning with the Pure Food and Drug Act of 1906, and strengthened by the 1938 Federal Food, Drug, and Cosmetic Act and subsequent amendments and decisions, the freedom of *informed* choice is well established, but there is no freedom to sell "snake oil" under false premises. Misrepresentation of facts in drug labeling and selling is a Federal offense. Attempts, for example, to designate Laetrile a vitamin (and thereby escape more stringent drug regulations) were struck down by the FDA (Food and Drug Administration, 1977).

In summary, health care practitioners have a responsibility to be sensitive to their patient's needs, to speak clearly when describing expectations, to look *into* people as well as *at* them and to treat them wisely and well. This approach will certainly increase effectiveness of patient-practitioner communication and trust, and thus assist in providing valuable guidance against the use of unproven methods.

CONCLUSIONS

The extent of quackery in cancer today is regrettably a reflection of inadequacy in the control of cancer by accepted methods, the inability of many to communicate with cancer patients, and the failure to provide support to the cancer patient and his family. To increase the credibility of providers and the effectiveness of the provision of health care, and thus to decrease the use of unproven therapies, it is essential that all health professionals develop an understanding of the psychosocial factors that propel patients toward unproven methods.

Practitioners should be conversant with the various unproven schemes and be prepared to discuss them with the patient openly and clearly. The patient must be told about his/her treatment and care, about the effects, outcomes, options and opportunities to participate in experimental protocols. The patient must be included in decision making and must be encouraged to participate in the process of getting well. This takes time and time must be offered by the provider to listen, to speak clearly, to explain to the family members, to discuss expectations, to indicate competence, to encourage, to allow expression of despair, fear and hopes, to establish belief in what the provider and the health care team have to offer and to indicate interest and understanding.

The patient and his or her family whose physician is unwilling to provide such information or to work with skilled and trained health care practitioners from other recognized fields, may not have an adequate physician. In this case the patient may be well advised to seek another opinion and if necessary, choose another doctor.

ADDITIONAL SOURCES OF INFORMATION

Information on unproven methods can be obtained from:

- *The American Cancer Society*. Look in the white pages for your nearest office.
- *Cancer Information Service* of the National Cancer Institute: Call 1-800-4-CANCER toll free.
- PDQ Information Center (A service which gives the physician access to all experimental protocols in the nation and provides listings of cancer specialists.) (301) 496-7403 or thru 1-800-4-CANCER.

REFERENCES

American Cancer Society, (1982, July). *Unproven Methods of Cancer Management*. Professional Education Publication No. 3014-PE. New York: American Cancer Society, Inc.

American Cancer Society. (1965, January 15). Medical Affairs Circular Letter MA-16.

American Cancer Society. (1984, April 6). Medical Affairs Circular Letter MA-17.

Barrett, S. (1980). *The Health Robbers. How to Protect Your Money and Your Life.* Philadelphia: George F. Stickley Co., p. 381.

Cassileth, B.R., Lusk, E.J., Strouse, T.B., & Bodenheimer, B. J. (1984). Contemporary unorthodox treatments in cancer medicine. A study of patients, treatments, and practitioners. *Ann Int Med* 101:105–112.

Consumer Reports. (1977, August). Laetrile: The political success of a scientific failure. Consumer Reports, pp. 444–447.

Curt, G.A. (1984). Warning on immunoaugmentative therapy. *N Engl J Med* 311:859.

Devesa, S.S. (1986). Cancer mortality, incidence, and patient survival among American women. *Women and Health* 11:7–22.

Doll, R., & Peto, R. (1981). The causes of cancer: Quantitative estimates of avoidable risks of cancer in the United States today. *JNCI* 66:1191–1308.

Food and Drug Administration. (1977, August 5). Laetrile: Commissioner's decision on status. *Federal Register* 42(151):39768–39806.

Funch, D.P. (1986). Socioeconomic status and survival for breast and cervical cancer. *Women and Health* 11:37–54.

Hach, J., & Wilson, S.A., (1986). Women and hospice care. *Women and Health* 11:155–163.

Herbert, V. (1984). Faddism and quackery in cancer nutrition. *Nutrition and Cancer* 6: 196–206.

Lowell, J. (1986). The Gerson Clinic. *Nutrition Forum* 3:9–12.

Moertel, C.G., Fleming, T.R., Rubin, J., Kvols, L.K., Sarna, G., Koch, R., Currie, V.E., Young, C.W., Jones, S.E., & Davignon, J.P. (1982). A clinical trial of amygdalin (Laetrile) in the treatment of human cancer. *N Engl J Med* 306:201–206.

Monaco, G. (1982). Countering health frauds. *Am J Pediatr Hematol/Oncol* 5(4):23–24.

National Council Against Health Fraud. (1984). *Unproven Methods of Cancer Management Surveillance Project Questionnaire.*

Penman, D., et al. (1986). The impact of mastectomy on self-concept and social function: A combined cross-sectional and longitudinal study with comparison groups. *Women and Health* 11:101–130.

Soskolne, C.L. (1986). Scientific and ethical conflicts in cancer studies involving human subjects. *Women and Health* 11:197–215.

Subcommittee on Unorthodox Therapies, American Society of Clinical Oncology. (1983). Ineffective cancer therapy: A guide for the layperson. *J Clin Oncol* 1:154–163.

Ulbricht, G.F. (1986). Laryngectomy rehabilitation: A woman's viewpoint. *Women and Health* 11:131–136.

Postmenopausal Estrogen, Cancer and Other Considerations

Elizabeth Barrett-Connor, MD

ABSTRACT. The female hormone estrogen is widely prescribed to postmenopausal women. Its major documented benefit is prevention of bone mineral loss, which is a major risk factor for fracture in the elderly. Its clearly documented risk is promotion of cancer of the endometrium. There is a growing body of data that suggests that postmenopausal estrogen therapy reduces the risk of cardiovascular disease. This benefit, if real, may be lost when a cyclic progestin is added to reduce the risk of cancer. Further studies are needed to provide a firmer basis for balancing these risks and benefits.

After the menopause, when ovarian estrogen and progesterone production has ceased, only a small amount of a relatively weak estrogen, estrone, is produced from adrenal androstenedione, conversion occuring primarily in adipose tissue. At the turn of this century, this estrogen deficiency did not matter: the average female in the United States did not reach the usual age of natural menopause; her life expectancy was not quite 50 years. In the 1980s, however, the average North American woman can expect to spend one-third of her life in the postmenopausal state; her life expectancy is nearly 80 years. As a consequence of this longer life expectancy, replacement estrogens might logically be prescribed for more years and for more women than ever before.

From the early 1960s to the mid 1970s postmenopausal estrogen prescription became very common in the United States, both to treat specific symptoms and to promote youth and health. The data presented here regarding the consequences of long term postmenopausal estrogen use come primarily from this country, such use having achieved far greater popularity in the United States than elsewhere.

Elizabeth Barrett-Connor is Professor and Chair, Department of Community and Family Medicine, University of California, San Diego, La Jolla, CA 92093.

Presented in part as the 14th Alexander D. Langmuir Lecture, Atlanta, GA, April 1985.

These data are particularly relevant to conjugated equine estrogen (Premarin), the most commonly prescribed estrogen in the United States, usually given in a dose of 0.625–1.25 mg without a progestin. The assumption that other estrogen preparations have similar risks or benefits is unwarranted, since the hormone potency of each may not be the same for the reproductive tract and other organs. Whether estrogens given with a progestin will have the same consequences as unopposed estrogen is discussed below.

Major known or possible risks and benefits of unopposed estrogen therapy include an *increased risk* of endometrial and breast cancer, and a *decreased risk* of osteoporosis and cardiovascular disease. Among these consequences, endometrial cancer has received the greatest attention but, as shown in Figure 1, is much less important than breast cancer or heart disease in terms of mortality. Myocardial infarction is by far the commonest cause of death in postmenopausal women at all ages. Although comparable data are unavailable for death due to osteoporotic fracture, the 12–20% excess mortality rates within one year of hip fracture almost certainly exceed those for endometrial cancer. Morbidity, as measured by hospitalization (Table 1), is also least for endometrial cancer, intermediate for breast cancer and hip fracture, and greatest for ischemic heart disease.

ENDOMETRIAL CANCER

Long before the estrogen-endometrial cancer association was first recognized, there were good reasons to suspect that estrogen could promote endometrial cancer. As long ago as 1941 estrogen was shown to cause endometrial cancer in an animal model, and more than 25 years have passed since it was clearly documentated that young women with estrogenic ovarian tumors have a high frequency of both endometrial hyperplasia and cancer. Postmenopausal overweight women are more prone to endometrial hyperplasia than their leaner peers and several case control studies have found an excess endometrial cancer risk in women with obesity or obesity-related conditions, such as diabetes and hypertension. This obesity-cancer connection is thought to be related to the higher levels of endogenous estrogen in postmenopausal overweight women.

Nevertheless, it was not until 1975 that an association of exogenous estrogen and endometrial cancer was first appreciated.

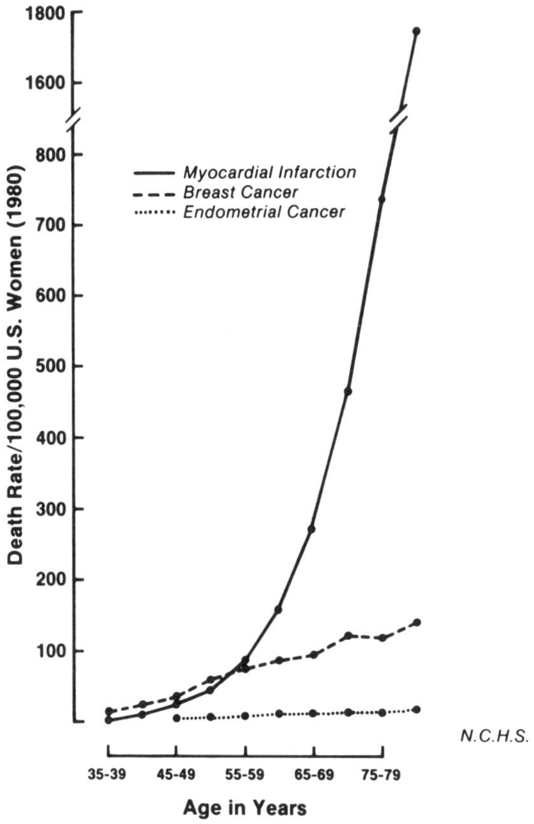

FIGURE 1. Myocardial infarction, breast cancer and endometrial cancer death rates in United States women. Data from National Center for Health Statistics, 1980.

Since then, estrogen-associated endometrial cancer has been labeled the largest iatrogenic epidemic of this century. It is certainly true that the incidence of endometrial cancer rose and fell in parallel with non-contraceptive estrogen prescription sales in the United States (while at the same time the incidence of endometrial cancer in women less than 50 years of age remained stable), and that more than twenty case control studies have now incriminated estrogen replacement therapy as a risk factor for endometrial cancer in postmenopausal women. Differences in the reported relative risk associated with extended estrogen use, shown in Table 2 for selected studies, probably reflect differences in selection or diagnostic criteria for cases

Table 1. U.S. Hospital Discharges by Diagnosis for Women Aged 55+ Years, 1983

DIAGNOSIS	NUMBER	RATE/1000	AVERAGE DURATION HOSPITAL STAY (DAYS)
Ischemic Heart Disease	752,000	26.6	9.2
Hip Fracture	165,000	5.8	17.6
Breast Cancer	165,000	5.9	10.0
Endometrial Cancer	37,000	1.3	9.4

National Hospital Discharge Survey; unpublished data kindly provided by NCHS.

Table 2. Estimated Relative Risks in Case-Control Studies of Endometrial Cancer and Postmenopausal Estrogen Use for Three or More Years.

FIRST AUTHOR (YEAR OF PUBLICATION)	NUMBER OF CASES	SOURCE OF CONTROLS	YEARS USE	ESTIMATED RELATIVE RISK
McDonald (1977)	145	Hospital	3	4.9
Hulka (1980)	186	Gynecology	3.5	4.1
Shapiro (1980)	149	Hospital	5	6.0
Jelovsek (1980)	431	Hospital	5	3.3
Antunes (1979)	451	Hospital	5	15.0
Ziel (1975)	94	Health Plan	7	13.9
Mack (1976)	63	Retirement Community	8	8.8
Kelsey (1982)	167	Hospital	7.6-10	8.2
Gray (1977)	205	Private Practice	10	11.6
Hoogerland (1978)	629	Hospital	10	6.7
Weiss (1979)	322	Community	11-14	24.2

Adapted from Brinton, 1984.

and controls, and in dose and duration of estrogen use in different study populations. Nevertheless, after considerable debate over methodologic issues, there is general agreement that unopposed postmenopausal estrogen (i.e., estrogen given without a progestin) promotes endometrial cancer, and that the risk increases with dose and/or duration of use. There is still disagreement on the duration of use required to show a significant excess risk (most studies say three years), the degree of relative risk (probably around 5–7 for the use of at least three years) and about how long risk persists after estrogen is discontinued.

Many studies have shown that estrogen-associated endometrial cancer is better differentiated, less invasive at diagnosis, and is less often fatal than endometrial cancer occuring in nonhormone using women. The mortality rate for endometrial cancer did not rise during the years when the incidence did, further evidence that the estrogen-associated cancer is not often fatal. Indeed, the mortality rate for women with estrogen-associated endometrial cancer may be less than that for women who had neither endometrial cancer nor estrogen-use. Nevertheless, the cancer risk cannot be ignored. Even a relatively benign cancer is an unacceptable complication of elective therapy unless an overriding benefit can also be documented.

OSTEOPOROSIS

If endometrial cancer is the best defined risk associated with extended estrogen replacement therapy, the prevention of osteoporosis is the best defined benefit. The association of endogenous sex hormones with osteoporosis was first appreciated in 1940, when Albright commented on the sex differential of osteoporosis and the frequency of bone loss following oophorectomy or natural menopause. Exogenous estrogens appear to improve calcium balance and may raise calcitonin levels, but it is still not clear how estrogens exert their protective effect. There are no known estrogen receptors in bone.

Because estrogen effects on bone can be demonstrated in as little as a month using absorptiometry or other sophisticated techniques, in the past ten years numerous clinical trials have been completed showing that estrogen can block the bone resorption that occurs after oophorectomy or natural menopause. Furthermore, bone mineral loss can be halted even when exogenous estrogen treatment is initiated several years after the menopause. Case-control studies confirm benefit; estrogen use is reported by more older women without fractures than by those with fractures (Table 3). Protection seems to be greatest when estrogens are begun soon after menopause and

Table 3. Estimated Relative Risks in Case-Control Studies of Hip and/or Wrist Fracture and Postmenopausal Estrogen Use

FIRST AUTHOR (YEAR OF PUBLICATION)	NUMBER OF CASES	DURATION OF USE	ESTIMATED RELATIVE RISK
Hutchinson (1979)	157	6 mo	0.68
Kreiger (1982)	98	6 mo	0.4-0.5
Paganini-Hill (1981)	91	1-60 mo	0.97
		61 mo	0.42
Weiss (1980)	320	1-2 yrs	0.84
		3-5 yrs	0.89
		6-9 yrs	0.38
		10 yrs	0.46

continued at least five years. Most women have no bone loss when taking 0.625 mg of Premarin (or 0.15 g of ethinyl estradiol), but higher doses may be better. In the case series of women with severe postmenopausal osteoporosis reported by Gordon et al., the subsequent vertebral fracture rate was significantly lower in those taking 1.25 mg vs. 0.6 mg of Premarin.

Once estrogen is stopped, bone loss resumes at the pretreatment rate. Much of the protective effect may be lost within a few years of discontinuing estrogen therapy. Nevertheless, Brody et al. calculate that postponing the onset of osteoporosis in postmenopausal white women by about five years would reduce their subsequent lifetime risk of hip fracture by about 50 percent.

BREAST CANCER

An association of endogenous estrogen with breast cancer risk is biologically plausible. As early as 1896 breast cancer regression was noted after oophorectomy; much later oophorectomized women were also found to be at lower risk of breast cancer. Other evidence compatible with an estrogen effect includes the sex ratio (breast cancer in men is rare, and often associated with exogenous estrogen), the well known and presumably endocrinologically mediated relation of breast cancer to reproductive history, the geographic differences in endogenous estrogen levels and breast cancer incidence, the demonstration of estrogen receptors in breast tissue, and the reports of lower levels of sex-hormone binding globulin in breast cancer patients.

Neither case control studies (Table 4) nor secular trend data, however, provide evidence that exogenous estrogens increase the risk of breast cancer. Neither dose nor duration of estrogen use has been consistently associated with increased breast cancer risk. Unfortunately only a few of the reported studies had a duration of estrogen treatment or followup that was longer than 7–10 years. Demonstration of an estrogen-breast cancer association might take longer; one study did find an increased risk of breast cancer in diethylstilbesterol (DES) users, but the association was not apparent until after 20 years. (The DES-breast cancer association, if real, may not apply to conjugated estrogens; DES is a different, non-steroidal compound and indications for its use could be markers for gonadal hormone abnormality and/or reproductive failure, which of themselves may be risk factors for breast cancer.)

In addition, it is always difficult to "prove" no association, and particularly so for a disease like breast cancer which has multiple

Table 4. Estimated Relative Risk from Ten Case-Control Studies of Breast Cancer in Women Who Ever Used Postmenopausal Estrogen.

FIRST AUTHOR (YEAR OF PUBLICATION)	NUMBER OF CASES	SOURCE OF CASES	SOURCE OF CONTROLS	ESTIMATED RELATIVE RISK
BCDSP (1974)	51	Hospital	Hospital	0.96
Craig (1974)	34	Population	Population	1.0
Casagrande (1976)	60	Population (?)	Doctors Office	0.75
	33	Population	Neighborhood	3.1
Sartwell (1977)	284	Hospital	Hospital	0.82
Ravnihar (1979)	177	Hospital	Hospital	0.73
Jick (1980)	97	Hospital	Hospital	0.97
Ross (1980)	131	Community	Community	1.1
Brinton (1981)	881	Screenees	Screenees	1.24*
Hoover (1981)	345	Population	Population	1.4*
Kelsey (1981)	332	Hospital	Hospital	0.9

*Borderline significance: lower 95% confidence limit equals 1.0

Adapted from Thomas, 1982.

putative risk factors that must be considered in the analysis. Very large samples are necessary to exclude an association: according to Arthes et al., in a case control study with a true hormone use history in 20%, 1400 cases and 1400 controls would be needed to give an 80% probability of detecting a true relative risk of 1.2.

Thus, although there is no evidence that exogenous estrogens increase the risk of breast cancer in the postmenopausal woman, limitations of sample size and duration of followup preclude a definitive statement.

CARDIOVASCULAR DISEASE

In most western countries the risk of ischemic heart disease is much lower in women than in men, and the sex differential is most notable before age 50. These observations led to the speculation that the favored status of premenopausal women is related to ovarian function. In support of this hypothesis are (1) animal models showing reduced atherosclerosis after exogenous estrogen or other maneuvers to "feminize" the estrogen/androgen ratio; (2) studies showing an increased risk of cardiovascular disease in oophorectomized women; and (3) studies of heart disease risk factors in postmenopausal women with and without estrogen replacement therapy, showing noncontraceptive estrogens have a favorable effect on lipoproteins and negligible effects on most other heart disease risk factors. Specifically, estrogen lowers LDL-cholesterol and raises HDL-cholesterol, primarily the HDL-2 subfraction that is most closely associated with protection.

Until recently, however, the possible cardiovascular benefit of estrogen therapy for postmenopausal women received little attention. This may have been a result of studies showing an excess of cardiovascular disease in estrogen-treated men and in oral-contraceptive-taking women. In both of these settings, the dose of estrogen usually exceeded that recommended for replacement estrogen; oral contraceptives also contain a progestin, which, as discussed below, may increase the risk of arterial disease.

As can be seen in Table 5, since 1974 many investigators have examined the relation of estrogen replacement therapy to cardiovascular disease risk in postmenopausal women, using different study designs and with diverse results. The majority of studies suggest that postmenopausal estrogen provides significant protection against

e.) In the prospective study of all cause *mortality* from
earch Clinics population, age-adjusted death rates in
g women were approximately half the rates in non-
aged 50 years and older. No evidence of bias favoring
nent of low risk women could be found, although there
n to expect that high socioeconomic status (low risk)
ose most likely to receive prescription for replacement
fore concluding overall benefit, however, it is impor-
er that there has been only one controlled clinical trial
randomly allocated to estrogen or placebo and with
wup (Table 6). That study, which did support overall
mall, restricted to women in a long term care hospital,
nformation is not given to evaluate the possibility that
were prescribed estrogen were healthier at outset, or
r medical care as a consequence.

PROGESTINS

orities, including the American College of Obstetrics
gy, have recommended that estrogen replacement ther-
with a progestin, in order to reduce the risk of endo-
. This recommendation has been widely accepted, in
unty 88% of practicing gynecologists surveyed gave a

en Year Followup of 84 Hospitalized Postmenopausal Women
andomly Assigned to Premarin (2.5 mg Daily) and
Provera (10 mg Daily x 7 d/mo) or Placebo

	TREATED	UNTREATED	P
s	4.8%	12.8%	0.05
ial	0	1.2	NS
	0	4.9	0.05
Infarction	1.2	3.7	NS
ebitis	15.5	18.3	NS
rtality	3.6	8.3	NS
Lipoprotein	0.883	0.982	0.05

chtigall et al., 1979.

Table 5. Estimated Relative Risk of Coronary Heart Disease in Women According to Postmenopausal Estrogen Use.

FIRST AUTHOR (YEAR OF PUBLICATION)	DESIGN(SIZE)	AGE IN YEARS POPULATION SOURCE	ENDPOINT	ESTIMATED RELATIVE RISK
Burch (1974)	historical cohort(737)	25 + one surgical practice	fatal coronary heart disease	0.43*
Rosenberg (1976)	case control (336)**	40-75 hospital patients	nonfatal myocardial infarction	0.47* (crude) 0.97 (adjusted)
Pfeffer (1978)	case control (185)	44 + retirement community	fatal and nonfatal myocardial infarction	0.68 (current use) 0.86 (ever use)
Jick (1978)	case control (17,19)	39-45 hospital patients	nonfatal myocardial infarction	7.5-9.3* (2 papers)
Gordon (1978)	prospective 24 yrs(")	40-54 Framingham community	coronary heart disease angina	1.6 2.3*
Nachtigal (1979)	double blind clinical trial 10 yrs (83 pairs)	mean age 55 chronic disease hospital patients	fatal and nonfatal myocardial infarction	0.33
Petitti (1979)	nested case control (26)	18-54 participants in contraceptive drug study	fatal and nonfatal myocardial infarction	1.2
Rosenberg (1980)	case control (447)	30-49 patients in coronary care units	nonfatal myocardial infarction	1.0 (recent use) 1.2 (past use)
Hammond (1979)	historical cohort(610)	age?; followed patients in university practice	incident cardiovascular disease	0.33*

Table 5 (continued)

FIRST AUTHOR (YEAR OF PUBLICATION)	DESIGN(SIZE)	AGE IN YEARS POPULATION SOURCE	ENDPOINT	ESTIMATED RELATIVE RISK
Ross (1981)	case control (133)	80 retirement community	fatal ischemic heart disease	0.43* (living controls) 0.57* (deceased controls)
Adam (1981)	case control (76)	50-59 decedents (one month) in England & Wales	fatal myocardial infarction	0.65*
Bain (1981)	nested case control (64)	33-55 nurses	nonfatal myocardial infarction	0.40* (oophorectomy) 0.70 (current users) 0.90 (ever users)
Szklo (1984)	case control (39)	35-64 hospital patients	nonfatal myocardial infarction	0.83 (crude) 0.61 (adjusted) 0.37 (surgical menopause)
Wilson (1985)	prospective 8 yrs (1234)	50-83 Framingham community	myocardial infarction angina pectoris	1.87 2.00*
Stampfer (1985)	prospective 4 yrs (32,317)	30-55 nurses	fatal and nonfatal coronary heart disease	0.30* (current use) 0.59 (past use)

* = p 0.05 ;** = number of cases

adapted in part from Bush and Barrett-Connor, 1985.

ischemic heart disease. The fe
are characterized by relative
women. The two case control
show a significantly increased
had low participation rates an
gen may variously increase
leading to hospitalization, it is
based on hospital-controls.)
studies, both derived from t
relative risk significantly gre
events exclusive of angina pe
as a marker for existing co
myocardial infarction in won

One of the most attractiv
heart-disease hypothesis is it
protein mechanism. This me
analyses: In Lipid Research
nificant protection is not app
multivariate model. The stud
lations specifically examined
trogen before and after HDL
Estrogen was associated with
that was independent of blood
cigarette smoking. When HD
of total cholesterol, most, b
estrogen disappeared. This a
much of its protective effect

ALL CAUSE MOR

In any speculation about r
issue is whether estrogen re
negative *overall* effect. No
excess overall morbidity and
opausal women compared to
amined several causes of *mor*
rates of several diseases; in t
reported to be significantly mo
taking estrogen compared to
confirmed, is biologically pla

are more acti
the Lipid Re
hormone-usi
using women
estrogen trea
is every reas
women are th
estrogens. B
tant to remen
with subjects
extended foll
benefit, was
and sufficien
women who
received bett

Several au
and Gynecol
apy be given
metrial canc
San Diego C

Table 6:

OBSERVAT

All Canc
Endome
Breast
Myocardi
Thrombop
Overall
Beta/Alp

Adapted from

progestin whenever they prescribed an estrogen for a postmenopausal woman with an intact uterus, as did at least 50% of family practitioners and internists. It is difficult to recall any other recent prophylactic drug regimen so widely accepted with so little critical study.

In the premenopausal woman, endogenous estrogen causes endometrial hyperplasia during the first half of the menstrual cycle; after ovulation and in the absence of pregnancy, this process is reversed by progesterone. Several studies have shown that progestins can prevent endometrial hyperplasia in post-menopausal estrogen-treated women, whereas cyclic estrogen does not. The optimal effect requires that progestin be given for at least 10 days each month. Because endometrial hyperplasia is a precursor of most cases of endometrial cancer, it is widely accepted that progestin would also prevent estrogen-associated endometrial cancer. At least one large case series, reported by Gambrell et al., supports this protective-effect hypothesis; women who received both estrogen and a progestin were at significantly lower risk of endometrial cancer than women who received estrogen alone. Unfortunately, data on obesity and other relevant covariates are not given for the women on each treatment regimen. Nevertheless, it is biologically plausible that progestin of adequate dose and duration can dramatically reduce the risk of endometrial cancer.

Progestin also does not interfere with the positive effect of exogenous estrogen in osteoporosis, and may even be complementary. A recent paper by Christiansen et al. partially supports earlier observations that estrogen plus progestin not only blocks bone loss but may lead to some bone mineral replacement.

Thus, progestin exerts a favorable effect with regard to the best documented risk of replacement estrogen (endometrial cancer) and does not reduce the best documented benefit (osteoporosis). Unfortunately, the facts with regard to breast cancer and heart disease are less simple and satisfactory.

In experimental models, progestins stimulate growth and proliferation of breast tissue to a far greater extent than estrogens. Although it is difficult to be sure that these studies used equivalent pharmacologic doses of the two hormones, these observations are at variance with the progestin-prevents-breast-cancer thesis. Gambrell has been the major supporter of the use of progestins to prevent breast cancer (and to improve the prognosis of patients who develop breast cancer). In his case series, women taking estrogen-progestin had significantly less breast cancer than women taking no gonadal hormones, as did women taking estrogen alone. If true, this work, and the only long term randomized clinical trial of estrogen—progestin vs. no hormone replacement (see Table 6), suggest that to prevent breast cancer combined estrogen plus progestin should be considered for all postmenopausal women, even those with hysterectomies. Unfortunately, neither paper provides sufficient information about the distribution of risk factors among women in each treatment group to be confident that the significantly lower risk of breast cancer is not due to substantial antecedent differences between treatment groups with regard to other risk factors. These data are certainly inadequate to recommend estrogen-progestin to reduce the risk of breast cancer.

Perhaps the most troublesome aspect of the progestin supplement to estrogen is with regard to heart disease. With the exception of the small clinical trial shown in Table 6, the long term cardiovascular risks and benefits of this regimen are unknown. As noted above, estrogen protection via the HDL mechanism is plausible and coherent with known facts. Progestins tend to block or reverse the favorable effect of estrogen on HDL-C and LDL-C. The 19 norprogestins with more androgenic properties are worse in this regard, but even the least androgenic progestin, medroxyprogesterone (Provera), at best masks the favorable effect of estrogen on lipoproteins. The increased risk of vascular disease in young women taking oral contraceptives, often cited as evidence that estrogens are harmful, is in fact more suggestive that progestins are noxious. Studies in the U.K. and Australia, where oral contraceptives containing fixed doses of synthetic estrogen and variable doses of progestin are used, show parallel increases in vascular disease risk and decreases in HDL-C with increasing progestin dose (Figure 2).

CONCLUSIONS

Estrogen-associated endometrial cancer may be completely prevented by the addition of a cyclic progestin, and progestin plus estrogen is at least as effective as estrogen alone with regard to osteoporosis. Weinstein has reviewed some of these data and concluded that *if* prevention of osteoporosis were the only benefit, extended use of unopposed postmenopausal estrogen would not be cost-effective but estrogen plus a progestin would be. This appar-

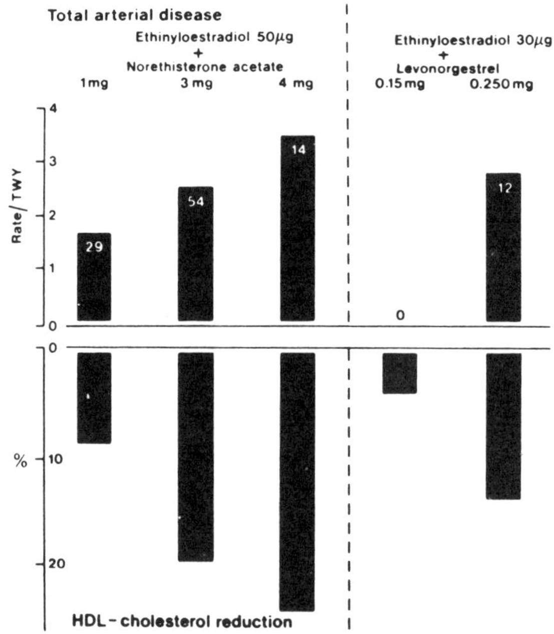

FIGURE 2. Rate of arterial disease (all types) per thousand women-years (TWY) and progestogen dose in five oral contraceptive products. Reproduced with permission from Kay, 1984.

ently happy solution is unfortunately not appropriate in the absence of better data about the long term effect of estrogen-progestin on all cause mortality, breast cancer and, particularly, cardiovascular disease.

REFERENCES AND SUGGESTED READINGS

Arthes, F., Sartwell, P., & Lewison, E. (1971, December). The pill, estrogens, and the breast. *Cancer*, Vol. 28, No. 6, 1391–1394.

Barrett-Connor, E., Brown, W. V., Turner, J., et al. (1979). Heart disease risk factors and hormone use in postmenopausal women. *JAMA*, 241, 2167–2169.

Brinton, L. (1984). The relationship of exogenous estrogens to cancer risk. *Cancer Detect Prev*, 7, 159–171.

Brody, J., Farmer, M., & White, L. (1984, December). Absence of menopausal effect on hip fracture occurrence in white females. *Public Health Briefs*, Vol. 74, No 12, 1397–1398.

Burch, J., Byrd, B., & Vaughn, W. (1975). The effects of long-term estrogen administration to women following hysterectomy. *Estrogens in the Post-Menopause. Front. Hormone Res.* 3, 208–214.

Bush, T., & Barrett-Connor, E. (1985). Noncontraceptive estrogen use and cardiovascular disease. *Epidemiol Rev*, 7, 80–104.

Bush, T. L., Cowan, L. D., Barrett-Connor, E., et al. (1983). Estrogen use and all-cause mortality; Preliminary results from the Lipid Research Clinics Program Follow-up Study. *JAMA*, 249, 903–906.

Chu, J., Schweid, A., & Weiss, N. (1982, July 1). Survival among women with endometrial cancer: A comparison of estrogen users and nonusers. *Am J Obstet Gynecol*, Vol. 143, No. 5, 569–573.

Collins, J., Allen, L., Donner, A., & Adams, O. (1980, November 1). Oestrogen use and survival in endometrial cancer. *The Lancet*, 961–964.

Christiansen, C., Nilas, L., Riis, B., Rodbro, P., & Deftos, L. (1985, October 12). Uncoupling of bone formation and resorption by combined oestrogen and progestagen therapy in postmenopausal osteoporosis. *The Lancet*, 800–801.

Cummings, S., Kelsey, J., Nevitt, M., & O'Dowd, K. (1985). Epidemiology of osteoporosis and osteoporotic fractures. *Epidemiol Rev*, 7, 178–208.

Elwood, J., & Boyes, D. (1980) Clinical and pathological features and survival of endometrial cancer patients in relation to prior use of estrogens. *Gynecol Oncol*, 10, 173–187.

Ernster, V., & Cummings, S. (in press). Communication re progesterone and breast cancer. *Obstet Gynecol*.

Fox, H. (1984). Endometrial carcinogenesis and its relation to oestrogens. *Path Res Pract*, 179, 13–19.

Gambrell, R. (1979). The role of hormones in the etiology of breast and endometrial cancer. *Acta Obstet Gynecol Scand*, Suppl., 88, 73–81.

Gambrell, R. Jr., Maier, R., & Sanders, B. (1983, October). Decreased incidence of breast cancer in postmenopausal estrogen-progestogen users. *Obstet Gynecol*, Vol. 62, No. 4, 435–443.

Gordan, G., Picchi, J., & Roof, B. (1973). Antifracture efficacy of long-term estrogens for osteoporosis. *Trans Assoc Am Physicians*, 86, 326–332.

Greenberg, E., Barnes, A., Resseguie, L. et al. (1984). A follow-up study of mothers exposed to diethylstilbestrol in pregnancy. *N Engl J Med*, 311, 1393–1398.

Hammond, C., & Maxson, W. (1982, January). Current status of estrogen therapy for the menopause. *Fertil Steril*, Vol. 37, No. 1, 5–25.

Hirvonen, E., Malkonen, M., & Manninen, V. (1981, March 5). Effects of different progestogens on lipoproteins during postmenopausal replacement therapy. *N Engl J Med*, Vol. 304, No. 10, 560–563.

Horsman, A., Jones, M., Francis, R., & Nordin, C. (1983, December 8). The effect of estrogen dose of postmenopausal bone loss. *N Engl J Med*, Vol. 309, No. 23, 1405–1407.

Hulka, B. (1980). Effect of exogenous estrogen on postmenopausal women: The epidemiologic evidence. *Obstet Gynecol Surv*, Supplement, Vol. 35, No. 6, 389–399.

Hutchinson, T., Polansky, S., & Feinstein, A. (1979, October 6). Post-menopausal oestrogens protect against fractures of hip and distal radius. *The Lancet*, 705–709.

Jick, H., Walker, A., & Rothman, K. (1980, March). The epidemic of endometrial cancer: A commentary. *AJPH*, Vol. 70, No. 3, 264–267.

Kay, C. (1984, December). The Royal College of general practitioners' oral contraception study: Some recent observations. *Clinics Obstet Gynaceol*, Vol. 11, No. 3, 759–786.

Kennedy, D., Baum, C., & Forbes M. (1985, March). Noncontraceptive estrogens and progestins: Use patterns over time. *Obstet Gynecol*, Vol 65, No. 3, 441–446.

Krauss, R., Lindgren, F., Wingerd, J., Bradley, D., & Ramcharan, S. (1978). Effects of estrogens and progestins on high density lipoproteins. *Lipids*, Vol. 14, No. 1, 113–118.

Kreiger, N., Kelsey, J., Holford, T., & O'Connor, T. (1982). An epidemiologic study of hip fracture in postmenopausal women. *Am J Epidemiol*, Vol. 116, No. 1, 141–148.

Lind, T., Cameron, E., Hunter, W., Leon, C., Moran, P., Oxley, A., Gerrard, J., & Lind,

U. (1979). A prospective, controlled trial of six-forms of hormone replacement therapy given to postmenopausal women. *Br J Obstet Gynecol*, Supplement 3, 1–29.

Lindsay, R., Hart, D., Forrest, C., & Baird, C. (1980, November 29). Prevention of spinal osteoporosis in oophorectomised women. *The Lancet*, 1151–1154.

Nachtigall, L. E., Nachtigall, R. H., Nachtigall, R. D., & Beckman, E. M. (1979). Estrogen replacement therapy. II. A prospective study in the relationship to carcinoma and cardiovascular and metabolic problems. *Obstet Gynecol* 54:74–79.

Paganini-Hill, A,. Ross, R., Gerkins, V., Henderson, B., Arthur, M., Mack, T. (1981). Menopausal estrogen therapy and hip fractures. *Ann Intern Med.* 95, 28–31.

Paterson, M., Wade-Evans, T., Sturdee, D., Thom, M., & Studd, J. (1980, March 22). Endometrial disease after treatment with oestrogens and progestogens in the climacteric. *Br Med J*, 822–824.

Schiff, I., Sela, H., Cramer, D., Tulchinsky, D., & Ryan, K. (1982, January). Endometrial hyperplasia in women on cyclic or continuous estrogen regimes. *Fertil Steril*, Vol. 37, No. 1, 79–82.

Shapiro, S., Kelly, J., Rosenberg, L., Kaufman, D., Helmrich, S., Rosenshein, N., Lewis, J., Knapp, R., Stolley, P., & Schottenfeld, D. (1985, October 17). Risk of localized and widespread endometrial cancer in relation to recent and discontinued use of conjugated estrogens. *N Engl J Med*, Vol. 313, No. 16, 969–972.

Stampfer, M., Willet, W., Colditz, G., Rosner, B., Speizer, F., & Hennekens, C. (1985, October 24). A prospective study of postmenopausal estrogen therapy and coronary heart disease. *N Engl J Med*, Vol. 313, No. 17, 1044–1049.

Thomas, D. (1982). Non-contraceptive exogenous estrogens and risk of breast cancer: A review. *Breast Cancer and Treat*, 2, 203–211.

Weinstein, M. & Schiff, I. (1983). Cost-effectiveness of hormone replacement therapy in the menopause. *Obstet Gynecol Surv*, Vol 38, No. 8, 445–455.

Weiss, N. (1983). Epidemiology of carcinoma of the endometrium. *Reviews in Cancer Epidemiology*, Volume 2, edited by Abraham M. Lilienfeld, 47–60.

Weiss, N., Ure, C., Ballard, J., Williams, A., & Daling, J. (1980). Decreased risk of fractures of the hip and lower forearm with postmenopausal use of estrogen. *N Engl J Med*, 303, 1195–1198.

Whitehead, M., Townsend, P., Pryse-Davies, J., Ryder, T., & King, J. (1981, December 31). Effects of estrogens and progestins on the biochemistry and morphology of the postmenopausal endometrium. *N Engl J Med*, Vol. 305, No. 27, 1599–1605.

Wilson, P., Garrison, R., & Castelli, W. (1985, October 24). Postmenopausal estrogen use, cigarette smoking, and cardiovascular morbidity in women over 50, the Framingham study. *N Engl J Med*, Vol. 313, No. 17, 1038–1043.

Scientific and Ethical Conflicts in Cancer Studies Involving Human Subjects

Colin L. Soskolne, PhD

ABSTRACT. Cancer studies involving human subjects present ethical conflicts which require a delicate balance to be struck between respect for fundamental human rights and the need to obtain sufficient data to satisfy study goals. Scientific and ethical conflicts at all stages of application of the scientific method are discussed. Legislative safeguards and ethical guidelines continue to evolve. Both must form an integral part of considerations regarding the feasibility of conducting cancer studies involving human subjects. Researchers, administrators, and legislators must be educated in and remain sensitive to two competing forces in epidemiologic research: the need to know versus respect for the individual's right to privacy, safety, dignity, and autonomy. An enhanced role for Institutional Review Boards to include an interactive monitoring function with ongoing studies is proposed.

INTRODUCTION

Selected scientific and ethical conflicts which relate to the epidemiological investigation of cancer are considered in this paper. The conflicts addressed pertain equally to cancers occuring in both sexes. However, the orientation is towards cancers occurring in women. The focus is on research involving human subjects as distinct from research in the basic sciences, *in vitro*, toxicologic, animal and other related cancer research.

Colin L. Soskolne is Associate Professor (Epidemiology), Department of Health Services Administration and Community Medicine, Faculty of Medicine, University of Alberta, Edmonton, Alberta, Canada. Address reprint requests to Dr. Soskolne at 13-103 Clinical Sciences Building, University of Alberta, Edmonton, Alberta, Canada T6G 2G3.

Professor Janet L. Storch reviewed earlier drafts of the manuscript and made many valuable comments for improvement to both the content and clarity of the presentation.

The manuscript was prepared by Ms. Treasure Whaley with her usual exceptional dedication and competence.

The scope of this paper is limited only to more current and topical conflicts, perceived by the author to be more recently recognized or more pressing than others. The scope is further narrowed to exclude records-based human studies, thus focusing more exclusively on those clinically-based research questions requiring direct human subject participation for their conduct. It should not be inferred that the issues discussed in this paper are of any greater or lesser importance than those topics not covered. The intent is to further stimulate discussion and thereby instill greater awareness of issues among all interest groups, including researchers and their subjects, physicians and their patients, high-technology industries, the pharmaceutical industry, ethics review boards, and legislators.

CANCER RESEARCH AND HUMAN SUBJECTS

1. Relationship Between Basic Sciences and Human Studies

Various types of research are undertaken to find the cause(s) of (the various) cancer(s), to identify improved early detection techniques, to test new treatment regimens (including surgery, chemotherapy, radiotherapy, and combinations of these), to test agents' primary and secondary prevention potential and to better identify high-risk groups for study purposes. The assumption in this massive enterprise is that disease can be prevented, and that early detection and appropriate therapies can result in reduced morbidity and in improved survival.

To remain relevant to human health, research undertaken in scientific laboratory settings is generally motivated by and justified in terms of observed human conditions. The utility of results from animal, bacterial or any other laboratory test systems must ultimately be tested in the human host before their effectiveness in human populations can be established. All branches of cancer research thus are interdependent, and contributions to knowledge emerge as a result of successful interactions among the various branches of scientific endeavor.

2. The Variety of Epidemiologic Approaches

There are various types of study designs in epidemiology which are used to test hypotheses and address specific scientific questions.

Some are based entirely on existing individual records, others require the linkage of existing individual records, and others require direct contact/communication with eligible research subjects. Some studies involve combinations of these approaches. The scope of this paper is limited to the situation of direct contact.

Studies involving direct contact with subjects may require a single contact or may require successive contacts over an extended period of follow-up and monitoring. The contribution of epidemiologic research to knowledge is directly related to the quality of data obtainable from human subjects. These data are often sensitive in nature, related to various lifestyle factors.

Trials involve subjecting one group of participants to one type of treatment and another group to a different treatment or to no treatment (i.e., a placebo). Trials often require stratification on potentially sensitive data and randomization, where the physician is excluded from decisions regarding the choice of therapy/intervention for his/her eligible patients.

3. *Patients and Subjects in Research*

From court rulings on U.S. Department of Health, Education and Welfare policy, a distinction was made between two types of individual participants in research involving human beings: patients and subjects.[1] With either, the researcher has an obligation to inform of both the risks and benefits associated with participation in research studies. In clinical-based cancer studies, physicians and other professionals serve the fundamentally important role of identifying eligible patients for accrual to trial. This requires the transfer of the patient to the status of subject and has been shown to create difficulties for the physician in terms both of informed consent and subsequent accrual to trial.[2–4]

The doctor-patient relationship has been investigated for many years. Dichter (1950),[5] even though addressing the physician as a caregiver (as opposed to a researcher), stressed the need for physicians to avoid the role of being directive (in full knowledge of his/her sense of power over the destiny of patients and any associated temptations), but rather to encourage autonomy as early in the relationship as possible. Mutual participation is viewed as maximizing the patient's autonomy and as being optimal in the management of chronic illness.[6] Autonomy thus may have a place not only in therapy, but also a corresponding role in research, particularly for obtaining informed consent from patients or subjects. However, barriers to the legal doctrine of informed consent do exist and form the subject of ongoing research.[2–4,7,8]

4. Modern Evolution of Ethical Conduct, the Law, and Their Influence on Participation

Since epidemiology generally depends for its conduct on the participation of those ill or those most at risk of becoming ill, the success of research today depends on the goodwill of people for their voluntary participation in research programs. The right to access existing records (whether individualized or aggregated), the right to approach the sick and/or the healthy to participate in research and the right of research participants to expect guarantees of data privacy are rights that have evolved and have been protected.[1,9] These rights have evolved since the Second World War with the recognition of the Nazi war crimes of the 1940s.[1] Human experimentation which had existed prior to the Nuremberg trials is no longer acceptable in most corners of the world.

As a direct consequence of the Nuremberg Code, experiments that in any way could endanger human life are done first in animal test systems and then, perhaps, in phase I trials on the terminally ill to determine, for example, toxic levels for subsequent drug therapy in less severely ill human subjects. When due confidence in the proposed therapy is attained, access to human subjects justifiably then may be gained. In turn, new therapeutic regimens/interventions then may be applied in the human context with the informed, voluntary participation of the human subject with due protection to the privacy interests of the subject.

Since 1974, with the introduction of the Privacy Act in the United States, [10] the major focus of legislation and subsequent investigative reports[11–14] is on the use of information gathered for one purpose—usually statutory reporting purposes—and its potential for use in other areas of interest. With distinct implications for the conduct of cohort and case-control studies in epidemiology, it bears little relevance to the protection of volunteer subjects in health interview settings where professional codes of ethical conduct (written or unwritten) define the nature of the relationship between the researcher and the study subject. Misconduct is dealt with through the professions' disciplinary bodies. The legislative process generally maintains a distance, and the timely resolution of professional misconduct is left to the professional societies.

No formal ethics guidelines exist specifically for the practitioners of epidemiology,[15] especially those who are not physicians; only implicit codes prevail. Researchers who are not governed by codes of ethical conduct and their subjects must be protected from any breach of trust. Invasion of privacy, as one breach of trust, could arise either by virtue of unscrupulous or unthinking researchers, or by the lack of formalized confidentiality requirements such as those that exist between physician and patient and which are duly respected by the law. Seriously jeopardized would be the potential for epidemiologic research if subjects had reason to believe that their data privacy were not guaranteed.[16,17]

Although institutions conducting research have established bioethics/research review committees—known more commonly as Institutional Review Boards (IRBs) in the U.S.A.—to preside over the ethical conduct of research administered within their institutions, legislative safeguards do not necessarily exist to protect participant privacy. IRBs continue to evolve[9] and in some jurisdictions, law also exists to protect the privacy of research participants. Laws, however, differ from one state or province within a country to another. Most recently, for example, California introduced legislation which protects subjects participating in AIDS-related research from any type of disclosure,[18] specifically disclosure related to human immunodeficiency virus antibody test results. It was found that such privacy safeguards were essential to ensuring participation goals for the conduct of epidemiologic research on human subjects, particularly where sensitive information is essential to the success of the study. Privacy is not only a fundamental human right, but it has to be especially protected for those people that make research possible by virtue of their voluntary participation. Since research is not above the law,[17] research that cannot guarantee privacy requires careful reconsideration.

SCIENTIFIC REQUIREMENTS FOR POPULATION STUDIES

Studies involving human subjects depend for their conduct on an observation or on a series of observations. Researchers are trained to put order into events that nature presents them with. "Whenever possible, the epidemiologist takes advantage of naturally occurring situations rather than undertaking an experiment.''[16] Because epidemiology often uses non-experimental methods applied to groups of people not monitored under laboratory conditions, standards commonly used in other branches of science may be violated in epidemiology owing to the use of more crude investigative procedures.[19] Violations can occur at the elementary level of data quality, choice of comparison group, and appropriateness of the methodology.[19] Hence, the need for the adequate documentation of epidemiologic research is essential if reviewers are to be able to assess data quality, the appropriateness of the methods used and evaluate any potential bias which may tend to support/invalidate the results.

SCIENTIFIC AND ETHICAL CONFLICTS

1. Perspectives

Conflicts between science and ethics arise at every step in our attempts to comply with the scientific method.[16] Since animal data cannot be assumed to apply in the human model, we are compelled to devise and conduct studies in human populations. These studies must neither infringe the rights of individuals nor impose any undue risks upon the participants. Such risks include not only physical harm associated with various therapies/interventions, but also more recently recognized potential psychological harm associated with participation in research,[20] as well as social harm associated with potential infringements of privacy.

Ensuring adherance to existing codes of ethical conduct will require continual education and vigilance by all groups concerned with the practice of epidemiologic research. While common practice guidelines applied by the researcher may always be called into question, the responsibility for their administration and implementation must remain not only with the researcher, but also with the IRB. As research hypotheses continue to become more refined, the balance between risks and benefits may become more delicate and less easily anticipated. Consequently, opportunities for the disregard of human rights in research may become too subtle to be identified early. Thus, the IRB and the researcher must interact to ensure conduct consistent with fundamental human rights. In turn, it is the IRB that must itself bear responsibility for protecting the study subject against any infringements to privacy from whatever source requests for information may come. Thus, it becomes important for legal safeguards to protect each of the human subject, the researcher, and the IRB.

Ethical conflicts that can arise within each step of the scientific method are described below.

2. Statement of the Problem, Ethics Justification and Participation

Some problems in cancer research may be intractable. Others may be more easily solved. Scientific ability may be attributed to those scientists who can identify problems not only worthy of epidemiologic investigation, but also capable of investigation. A problem both worthy and capable of investigation would be one built on existing scientific evidence with the justifiable intent of further advancing knowledge. Thus, when a problem is posed for further research, it should be scientifically defensible. In addition, its solution must be reasonably certain; false promises to advance knowledge would be unethical. Human studies designed to produce equivocal results would be unethical, but would not likely be approved for financial support or on moral grounds.

Susser et al., (1978),[16] draw attention to the motivation for selected research questions: "The choice of a research question raises broad issues. New knowledge is assimilated . . . within the bounds of dominant scientific paradigms that are, in turn, dependent on the social structure and values of the time." Assessment of relevance is in the hands of granting agencies where mode of functioning raises problems of values, political, moral and scientific, which are bound to have ethical implications.[16]

It may be argued that there are degrees of severity in ethics. Studies involving only existing records may have less potential for ethics infringements (i.e., harm to the individual) than studies subjecting healthy participants to (chemoprevention) trials.[21] In the latter situation, one may ask whether the stated problem is defensible in the context of prior scientific knowledge. The potential for personal harm to the subject is evident in the situation where drugs may be administered in the absence of support for the safety of such drugs in human populations.[16] The degree of ethics violation no doubt is related to both the specific cancer and the study design. The dilemma for the researcher and the IRB is to weigh the potential for individual harm against potential benefits to be gained.

Although notifiable disease legislation is often associated with sexually transmitted diseases, cancer also is reportable in some jurisdictions. In other jurisdictions, cancer reporting is encouraged and is protected under the law; cancer registries and reporting agencies are protected under cancer-related legislation. The protection usually pertains, however, only to existing registry records-based research studies.

In those instances where direct contact with eligible subjects is necessary for the conduct of a research study, not only is IRB clearance usually a requirement, but the informed consent and voluntary participation of each individual eligible research subject is negotiated between the researcher and the research subject. At that time, informed consent would include notice that under exceptional circumstances, records may be subpoenaed. However, this warning may not always be required in the consent form, since attributes recorded in research studies may not be perceived to be in the realm of potential questions of litigation when the study is designed. Questions regarding right of access, even under subpoena, would then raise important ethical questions, particularly if the justification for the subpoena arose through legislative changes promulgated after the initiation of the research. In those instances where risk of subpoena was omitted from the consent form in error, the researcher and the IRB should defend the privacy of every participant. Failure to do so might risk the continuation of the research program, unless every subject is successfully called back to sign an amendment to the consent document and agrees to such an amendment.

Individuals may be identifiable through rosters of individualized records created in the research process. Given that access may be required under the law, the expectation is that the key to such access would be by individual name rather than by a search of the data base on a set of particular characteristics. The identification of individuals with certain recorded attributes is always possible through a computerized or manually operated data bank. Potential access to research data by law enforcement agencies makes the conduct of epidemiologic research, particularly in those areas dealing with sensitive (e.g., sexual activities) and/or illegal acts (e.g., drug abuse) difficult, if not impossible. The conflict stems from the scientific need to know, the individual's right to privacy, and the common good. To minimize potential conflicts, assurances that respect the subjects' right to privacy must be entrenched, lest an action occurs that exposes research participants. Infringements of privacy could serve to undermine the goodwill and trust that must exist between the researcher and the study subject. No agency (government or otherwise) should, in these research circumstances, be permitted access to rosters of research participants in any society that professes to adhere to principles of fundamental human rights despite any legal issues associated with the data collected.

While it must remain true that research studies are not above the law, any breach of confidence required under the law would serve as a barrier to all future communications between the researcher and the subject.[17] To avoid such eventualities, research questions should be confined to those domains not in potential conflict with the law. For example, sexual histories should not be sought from adults regarding partners under the age of 16 years, since this would obligate the researcher to report the subject to child welfare authorities in many jurisdictions. On the other hand, where the research question was of sufficient importance, the law ought to protect both the subject and the researcher. The potential for successful research will be dramatically reduced if researchers are perceived as an exploitable resource for law enforcement or even for public health agencies. Every precaution must be taken to ensure that research can be conducted, unfettered by law or government in terms of protecting the privacy of research subjects.

3. *Specification of Hypotheses to be Tested*

The major hypotheses to be investigated in any study could be intended either to break new scientific ground or to replicate formerly generated discoveries. Since the statement of the problem is a necessary prerequisite to the specification of the hypotheses, we will assume that if the statement of the problem is both ethically and scientifically sound, then the objectives of the study as specified through the hypotheses to be tested, in turn, will be sound. However, if the objectives/hypotheses that are specified are not feasible in terms of data adequacy, sample size, and statistical power considerations, then the conduct of a study not capable of rendering results (i.e., incapable of advancing scientific knowledge), may be deemed unethical.

The scientific method would require that the hypotheses be testable prior to initiating the study. Otherwise, expending public resources on such research and the exploitation of the public's goodwill in terms of voluntary participation, may be perceived as having been solicited under false pretenses and would hence be deemed unethical. Thus, the question of feasibility is important both for the scientific intent of the study and for the ethical implications to the study subjects whose voluntary participation is to be sought. Questions of relevance, however, are not always as obvious or clear cut; they can often be influenced by the realities of available funding and political will.[16]

Chemoprevention research embraces the area of non-therapeutic drug research, usually requiring healthy human subjects for its conduct. While the benefits to society of well-conducted, non-therapeutic research are potentially great, what moral duty should society bear to compensate study subjects injured in society's own best interest?[22] Weed (1983)[22] believes that not only should a monetary award be made in direct relation to the severity of any untoward harm that befalls a study subject, but also that everything necessary from a medical/surgical perspective should be done to restore the individual to his/her prior state of health. These agreements should be incorporated into the consent document.[22] The tasks of adjudication of present and past health and of what medical/surgical procedures indeed are possible, are duties that IRBs will need to assume, or to assign. If the IRB deems that potential benefits outweigh potential risks (including costs through compensation)—based on a well-and-feasibly designed study—then approval may be granted.

More generally, "whether it is ethical to undertake a clinical trial is related to beliefs regarding the risks or benefits of a new treatment."[16] Bradford Hill (1962)[23] argued that it is unethical *not* to conduct a controlled trial of a new and untested treatment prior to its adoption for common usage. In yet other circumstances, "the social and scientific climate may precipitate a clinical trial before the safety of the agent has been satisfactorily demonstrated in animal experiments."[16] In addition, the withholding of a treatment that is untried but is believed by some to be efficacious presents as another ethical issue. Opinion prevailing at the initiation of a trial that the "untreated" group is at a disadvantage, and thus exposed to undue risk, has many times been stultified when put to trial.[16] Each scenario presents ethical dilemmas in conflict with the scientific method.

4. The Experimental Method and Informed Consent

Epidemiologic methodology incorporates questions both of study design and biostatistical techniques for data analysis. The study design must be appropriate to the hypothesis to be tested. In turn, the statistical methods must be appropriate to the study design for the production of true results. From a moral viewpoint, it would be inappropriate to recruit human subjects into a study for which neither the design nor the analytic techniques were proper.

Included under methodology we may consider questions of informed consent in relation to participant eligibility, particularly for those studies requiring direct participant contact. We might presume that if a problem has been appropriately stated, the hypotheses clearly specified, and the design and analytic techniques properly substantiated, then any problems pertaining to the participation of human subjects would be minimal. Yet, in studies involving the randomization of patients, the willingness of physicians in primary, secondary, or tertiary care practice is crucial to their success.[2–4,7,8] Participating physicians, particularly those in collaborative multicenter trials, are depended upon for their identification of eligible subjects and for negotiating with their patients questions of optimal therapy/intervention. The goal is to accrue patients to trial.

Since informed consent requirements are different around the world, their application cannot be expected to be standard. In addition, since the patient's dependence upon the physician for guidance also varies around the world, it might be expected that different types of patients likely will be randomized to trial in different countries. For example, physicians practicing in environments where paternalism[24,25] in decision-making is the norm, will have greater control over potentially less-informed human subjects. In environments where informed consent requirements are stringently applied, physicians may be less easily able to accrue patients to trial when having to justify decisions in the presence of therapeutic uncertainties. In differing cultural contexts then, physicians may perceive their role in relation to their patients differently. The impact of such potential differences on the results of randomized controlled trials in terms of biases that could exist, requires ongoing investigation.

The scientific method would dictate that eligible participants for a trial be randomized. However, in practice, interpersonal interactions in a cultural context might serve to undermine the recruitment goals of a particular study. The ethical conflict that arises stems from the physician's role as a caregiver as opposed to that of the physician who is more of an experimentalist. One might expect the physician inclined towards experimentation to randomize a greater proportion of his/her patients to trial as opposed to the physician inclined towards the role of a therapist. In addition, accrual of only selected patients to trial by physicians who do not feel they can adhere to strict codes of eligibility and subsequent randomization, leads to biases that undermine both the interpretation and generalizability of a trial. Further investigation into the behavioral aspects of the investigator-patient relationship was previously noted as being particularly pressing, since fear of change in this relationship was the most common reason given for not entering eligible patients into a trial of surgery for breast cancer.[2] "The role, values, and interests of the researcher, whether epidemiological or clinical, are different from those of the professional providing care, even when combined in the same individual."[16]

In a more recent study of physician opinions concerning informed consent, physicians believed that verbal consent would be adequate, providing greater opportunity for the physician to apply discretion to tailor the informed consent to suit individual needs.[8] It is apparent that physicians are being required to perform a function that may be incongruent with their training and perceived role as caregivers.[7,8] The difficulty of separating the perceived physician-patient and physician-subject roles[1] is evident in this conflict.

5. *Expectation as a Basis for Comparison*

Predicting the effect of an experimental treatment or intervention forms the basis for determining minimum sample size requirements. Selecting an appropriate or fair basis for comparison against which an effect is to be assessed, is recognized not only as being difficult to achieve, but as the "hallmark of the scientific experiment."[19] The choice of comparison group is fundamental to establishing observational or experimental effects, and hence has significant ethical underpinnings.

Experimental epidemiology, involving randomization and double-blind procedures eliminates, or at least reduces to a minimum, any potential bias between the groups being compared. It is thus the method of choice, provided that due justification can be provided (including questions of ethics) for a randomized controlled trial.

6. Analysis and Inference

Scientific researchers—practitioners of science—are assumed to have had adequate training in those analytic techniques appropriate to the nature of their data and the design of studies. It is incumbent upon the educational institutions that produce researchers to ensure that the graduate students capable of conducting research. Such students must be aware of their strengths and weaknesses; in areas where they are weak, it is incumbent upon them to bring together a team of colleagues that complements the abilities of all team members. Alternatively, expertise may be bought through consultant advisors. Regardless of the approach, no research activity should be supported which cannot show the requisite degree of competence in all necessary areas. In addition, graduating students should have been formally exposed to questions of morality and ethics in science.

Any conclusions drawn from the data analysis should not extend beyond the limits of the data and, where speculation is adopted, this should be clearly indicated in the preparation of a resulting manuscript. Ethical conflicts can arise when the interpretation of data extends beyond the limits of the data without reference to such inferences as being speculative on the part of the author.

7. The Documentation of Research Findings

The scientific method dictates the accurate recording of experimental observation. The meticulous recording and subsequent storage and retrievability of research data is that component of research which facilitates subsequent analysis. The scientific method also dictates the formal documentation of all methods utilized in the study; in most instances, the description of the methods should facilitate the replication of the study by other researchers as well as an assessment of the extent of any potential bias that might strengthen or weaken the findings of the study.[19] Ethical and moral conflicts can arise in those instances where deliberate omissions or amendments to the methods are documented, different from those actually used.

It is not surprising that when a carefully designed and executed study is completed, the researcher would wish it to be published. Publication, after all, exposes the work to extensive review and is an important criterion for upward mobility in the research labor market. Yet, attention has been drawn to two types of error that can arise when decisions are made about publication: the results of a study could be false and should not be accepted for publication, or results that could be true are not accepted for publication.[26] In the absence of knowledge about the truth, however, great care thus needs to be exercised in both the research itself and, in particular, assessment of bias or any consideration that may provide evidence to invalidate the findings. Usually, however, assessments are likely to modify results rather than render them unpublishable. "The dilemma is how to make the best decisions about when to publish, and when to refrain from doing so . . . The risk of error imposes the need for responsible behavior."[26] This pertains especially in the field of applied science, perhaps most conspicuously in the epidemiology of drug effects, where erroneous findings potentially can have a relatively rapid direct impact on morbidity and mortality. An ethical conflict thus exists between the need for scientific knowledge, the publish or perish ethic, and the potential interpretation and utilization of published findings. Perhaps a greater focus needs to be placed on understanding the results of epidemiologic studies, especially regarding constraints on their interpretation,[27] rather than on limiting those publications which well may contribute to the advancement of epidemiology.

It is not unknown in science for scientists to use dishonest means to establish themselves and further their careers.[28,29] Pressures to publish have been cited as one possible cause for dishonesty in science. Other reasons, including those associated with ego, overzealousness, and vested interests, have been presented in recent chronicles that document history of fraud and deceit in the halls of science. A text by Broad and Wade, 1985,[29] is so powerful in its ability to raise awareness about misconduct in science that it should form part of the educational requirements for all aspiring scientifically oriented individuals.

CONCLUSIONS AND RECOMMENDATIONS

Questionable ethical conduct arises when a decision, pertaining to the application of the scientific method in the context of human subjects, is made based on either unintentional error or with premeditated intent. Unintended error could be based on lack of training, lack of experience or an oversight and should be detectable through the review process. Premeditated error, however, is likely to be more difficult to detect. Either type of error will be more difficult to detect, the more refined and subtle the distinctions being hypothesized and tested.

It has been suggested that the institutional-administrative response to misconduct in science might somehow be accelerated in order to remove false leads and minimize their impact on the advancement of knowledge.[28,29] Mechanisms to achieve such an accelerated response need to be explored and implemented.[28] Many scientific associations, societies, and organizations have initiated the development of codes of ethical conduct for their membership.[15] The underlying objective in the establishment of such codes is to imbue scientists in the many disciplines associated with the advancement of science, with a set of moral and ethical principles that will maximize adherance to the scientific method and minimize the practice of fraud and deceit in science. Some scientific bodies also have developed disciplinary mechanisms for the handling of fraud and deceit among their membership. More recently, others have developed codes specific to cancer centers.[30]

Since epidemiologic research, by its nature, has to investigate diseases where they occur, prevailing social values as expressed through legislation and legislative enforcement, should include both an appreciation and a respect for those individuals that participate in research, if knowledge is to be advanced. To expect the voluntary participation of the ill and even of healthy (control) subjects, researchers must be in the strongest possible position to provide assurances as to the right to privacy of the participant; assurances that rights will not be infringed should be clear both to the researchers and the study participants *prior* to embarking on studies involving human subjects. The privacy of all data collected on individuals must be guaranteed and respected. In the absence of such guarantees, it is likely that willingness of eligible people to participate in research will decline and the potential to derive benefit for the common good would be reduced significantly. Without willing study subjects, epidemiologic knowledge cannot be advanced because the nature and extent of problems that could otherwise be studied would be limited as a function of the perceived sensitivity of the personal data requirements for the contemplated research.

It is clear that the degree of sophistication of IRBs, in terms of risk-benefit-value considerations, will by necessity have to grow. Caution has been raised, however, against the introduction of further regulations to ensure the ethical conduct of trials. While recognizing the moral basis that protects the rights of study subjects in the western world, concern has been expressed that over-regulation can "damage the fragile structure of this important area of research (i.e., clinical investigation) without contributing significantly to the preservation of human dignity."[31] Over-regulation which makes the enrollment of participants to trial an impediment, must be avoided, lest potentially important studies be discouraged. To facilitate accrual and participation, however, government may need to entrench legislation which limits access to research data, in whole or in part, particularly by subpoena. A two-step process may be desirable: (i) a public airing of all interests (including the risk-benefit for research), followed by (ii) a majority vote by government, analogous to constitutional amendment requirements, for access to research data. Only then may sufficient confidence prevail for the protection of individual privacy, so fundamental to the success of meeting recruitment goals for epidemiologic research. In addition, "the IRB system will continue to evolve to better balance burdens on investigators and protection of subjects."[32]

Clearly, ethical dilemmas contribute to making research a slow evolutionary process. Despite the ethical issues that arise in the conduct of research, sight must not be lost of those ethical issues that are spawned in the absence of research. It is important to consider the question relating to the ethics of caregivers who administer treatments/interventions in the *absence* of supporting scientific evidence.[23,33] The administration of "care" based on faith rather than evidence indeed may continue to parallel scientific advance until such time as more defensible research protocols can be advanced. The basis for such faith, however, must be subjected to ongoing evaluation.

In those research endeavors where risk and benefit are either not specifiable or are specifiable but in proportions not acceptable to IRBs, research may need to be halted. The time well may have arrived or soon be upon us where the dignity of the human subject and our concerns for both morality and ethics have to outweigh our determination to contribute to the continued advance of knowledge and hence of human health. Perhaps only when the subjects' basic human values can be accommodated in the formulation of the risk-benefit equation should volunteers be recruited to trial; in life-threatening situations, participation in a trial may be more acceptable than among the healthy. However, trials confined to selected volunteers are of limited generalizability, and may be of little or no consequence in the area of primary and even secondary prevention. In particular, trials whose recruitment and participation success depends on financial compensation/reward as an inducement, may further limit the generalizability of research findings and may be viewed further as being "inherently coercive."[34]

In a recent paper, patient autonomy is given major emphasis in determining how much the cancer patient should know and decide: "The guiding principle is respect for persons, which means that competent patients have the right to know and to decide . . . Consent that is not informed is not valid; it does not give clinicians a right to proceed with diagnostic or therapeutic procedures."[35] While these guiding principles have been conceptualized in the context of the cancer patient, these principles have been extended to clinical trials: "Concern for the interests of the subject must always prevail over the interests of science and society."[36] The primacy of the physician-patient relationship has been stressed in that only if the physician believes that the participation of the patient in a trial is in the patient's best interest, then the physician ought to encourage—indeed, urge—such participation.[36] Thus, the distinction between patient and subject has been made,[1,36] wherein the informed consent process in research (by its nature) differs greatly from that in medical practice. It then becomes paramount for the success of trials, for cancer specialists to be convinced of the potential contribution of the trial to knowledge relative to existing uncertainties if their indispensible role in the accrual of patients/subjects is to be effective.

NOTES

1. Gray, B.H. (1975). *Human subjects in medical experimentation: A sociological study of the conduct and regulation of clinical research.* New York: John Wiley & Sons.

2. Taylor, K.M., Margolese, R.G., & Soskolne, C.L. (1984). Physicians' reasons for not entering eligible patients in a randomized clinical trial of surgery for breast cancer. *The New England Journal of Medicine, 310*, 1363–1367.

3. Kelsey, J.L. (1981). Privacy and confidentiality in epidemiological research involving patients. *IRB: A review of human subjects research, 6*, 1–4.

4. Singer, E. (1980). More on the limits of consent forms. *IRB: A review of human subjects research, 2*, 7.

5. Dichter, E. (1950). *A psychological study of the doctor-patient relationship.* California Medical Association.

6. Enelow, A.J., & McKinney, L. (1979). Basic Interviewing. In *Interviewing and patient care.* (2nd ed.) pp. 35–61, Enelow, A.J. & Swisher, S.N. (Eds.). New York: Oxford University Press.

7. Lidz, C.W., Meisel, A., Osterweis, M., Holden, J.L., Marx, J.H., & Munetz, M.R. (1983). Barriers to informed consent. *Annals of Internal Medicine, 99*, 539–543.

8. Taylor, K.M., Shapiro, M., Soskolne, C.L. & Margolese, R.G. (1986). A mixed blessing. Physicians' interpretation of informed consent for randomized breast cancer trials. (In preparation).

9. Hosford, B. (1986). *Bioethics committees: The health care provider's guide*. Rockville, MD: Aspen System Corporation.

10. Privacy Act of 1974. Establishment of system records. *Federal Register*, Monday, July 25, 1983, 48(143):33748–51. Washington, DC: Government Printing Office.

11. Task Force on Environmental Cancer and Heart and Lung Disease. (1984). *Legal and administrative impediments to the conduct of epidemiologic research*. U.S. Environmental Protection Agency: Pavlova, M., & Young, P.

12. U.S. Congress. House subcommittee on oversight and investigations of the committee on interstate and foreign commerce. (1980). *Data transfer restrictions impede epidemiologal research*. 96th Congr., 2nd sess.

13. U.S. Department of Health & Human Services. (1980). *Environmental Health: A plan for collecting and coordinating statistical and epidemiologic data*. DHHS Publication No. (PHS) 80–1248. November 4, 1983. Washington, DC: Government Printing Office.

14. U.S. Department of Health & Human Services. (1981). Data systems of the National Center for Health Statistics. In *Vital and Health Statistics*. Series I Programs and Collection Procedures, No. 16. DHHS Publication No. (PHS) 82–1318. Washington, DC: Government Printing Office.

15. Soskolne, C.L. (1985). Epidemiological research, interest groups and the review process. *Journal of Public Health Policy, 6*, 173–184.

16. Susser, M., Stein, Z., & Kline, J. (1978). Ethics in epidemiology. *Annals of the American Academy of Political & Social Science, 437*, 128–141.

17. Fetterman, D.M. (1984). Guilty knowledge, dirty hands, and other ethical dilemmas: The hazards of contract research. In *Ethnography in educational evaluation.*, D.M. Fetterman (Ed.). California: Sage Publications, Inc.

18. CAL. Health Code Section 199.20, 1985.

19. Feinstein, A.R. & Horwitz, R.I. (1982). Double standards, scientific methods, and epidemiologic research. *The New England Journal of Medicine, 307*, 1611–1617.

20. Loftus, E.F. (1979). Informed consent may be hazardous to your health. *Science, 204*, editorial.

21. Gordis, L., Gold, E., & Seltser, R. (1977). Privacy and protection in epidemiologic and medical research: Challenge and responsibility. *American Journal of Epidemiology, 105*, 163–168.

22. Weed, D.L. (1983). Ethics and chemoprevention research. *Seminars in Oncology, X*(3), 355–359.

23. Bradford Hill, A. (1962). *Statistical methods in clinical and preventive medicine*. New York: Oxford University Press.

24. Childress, J.F. (1982). *Who should decide? Paternalism in health care*. New York: Oxford University Press.

25. Gillon, R. (1985). Paternalism and medical ethics. *British Medical Journal, 290*, 1971–1972.

26. Shapiro, S. (1985). The decision to publish. Ethical dilemmas. *Journal of Chronic Diseases, 38*, 365–373.

27. Block, G., & Hartman, A.M. (1983). Understanding the results of epidemiologic studies. *Seminars in Oncology, X* (3), 257–263.

28. Petersdorf, R.G. (1986). The pathogenesis of fraud in medical science. *Annals of Internal Medicine, 104*, 252–254.

29. Broad, W. & Wade, N. (1985). *Betrayers of the truth*. London: Oxford University Press.

30. van Eys, J., Bowen, J.M., Alt, J. et al. (1986). Creating a code of ethics: Report of

the University of Texas System Cancer Center M.D. Anderson Hospital and Tumor Institute. *Ca-A Cancer Journal for Clinicians, 36*, 115–119.

31. Cooper, B.A. (1985). Clinical investigation under attack: The threat of over-regulation. *Future Health*. Winter, 7–8.

32. Robertson, J.A. (1981). Legal considerations in clinical cancer research. *Seminars in Oncology, VIII*(4), 442–446.

33. Lacher, M.J. (1981). Patients and physicians as obstacles to a randomized trial. *Seminars in Oncology, VIII*(4), 424–429.

34. Wikler, D. (1981). Ethical considerations in randomized clinical trials. *Seminars in Oncology, VIII*(4), 437–441.

35. Schoene-Seifert, B. & Childress, J.F. (1986). How much should the cancer patient know and decide? *Ca-A Cancer Journal for Clinicians, 36*, 85–94.

36. Levine, R.J. (1986). Referral of patients with cancer for participation in randomized clinical trials: Ethical considerations. *Ca-A Cancer Journal for Clinicians, 36*, 95–99.

Women, Smoking, Cigarette Advertising and Cancer

Virginia L. Ernster, PhD

ABSTRACT. Cigarette smoking is a major cause of cancer in women, accounting for about one-fourth of their estimated 219,000 cancer deaths per year. Cigarette smoking specifically increases a woman's risk of developing cancer of the lung, larynx, esophagus, oral cavity, pancreas, kidney, bladder, and possibly uterine cervix. During the past twenty years, concerted efforts have been made by the tobacco industry to increase sales to women. Strategies have included development of "feminine" brands such as Virginia Slims, slick media campaigns portraying smoking as elegant and glamorous, and sponsorship of fashion, women's sports events, and even medical programs. Reversal of these alarming trends requires that women as well as men recognize the role of cigarette smoking in cancer causation, and support programs which promote non-smoking as well as combat the influence of the tobacco industry on women's smoking behavior.

"I'm a nonsmoker, so information on smoking isn't relevant to me."

"I'm a smoker and I know I should quit, so stop bugging me."

It is difficult to package the subject of smoking in an appealing way. Nonsmokers understandably feel the issue doesn't apply to them, and smokers resent being told what to do. Most people know that smoking is not a healthy behavior, and smoking is becoming increasingly unpopular in the U.S., with smoking prevalence figures declining each year. Continued attention to smoking is necessary, however, because the full magnitude of its attendant health risks is

Virginia L. Ernster is with the Department of Epidemiology and International Health, School of Medicine, University of California at San Francisco, San Francisco, CA 94143.

This article was supported in part by USPHS grant P01 CA 13556-14 from the National Cancer Institute, Bethesda, MD.

generally not appreciated, particularly among smokers. One in three Americans continues to smoke cigarettes, and tobacco remains an extremely profitable product.

Why is smoking a special issue for women? In terms of cancer risk, the answer is simple: smoking contributes to at least one in four cancer deaths among American women,[1] a proportion that is expected to continue to increase as cohorts characterized by heavy smoking age. Moreover, smoking rates among women—unlike men—have declined only slightly. Tragically, lung cancer has surpassed breast cancer to become the leading cause of cancer death in American women. Were it not for trends in smoking-related cancers, most notably the epidemic of lung cancer, age-adjusted overall cancer rates in American women would be declining much more dramatically than is currently the case.

This paper first summarizes the relationship of smoking to a variety of cancers in women and, second, discusses the wide range of cigarette brands, advertisements and other promotions targeted to women. It concludes with a discussion of recommended actions for health professionals and consumer groups to reduce the prevalence of smoking and, ultimately, the incidence of cancer in American women.

SMOKING AS A RISK FACTOR FOR CANCER

Cigarette smoking increases the risk of cancer of many sites, including lung, larynx, esophagus, oral cavity, bladder, kidney, pancreas and cervix. The strength of the relationship differs across sites, being especially marked for lung cancer. The evidence for each site is summarized briefly below.

Lung Cancer

Lung cancer mortality rates among women in the United States have increased dramatically since 1950. That year, lung cancer ranked seventh among cancer causes of death in women, accounting for only about 3% of female cancer mortality.[2] By 1985, lung cancer surpassed breast cancer to become the leading cause of cancer death in American women, accounting for 18% of all female cancer deaths.[3] Allowing for an appropriate lag time, the increase in lung cancer rates paralleled the increases in female smoking prevalence that began in the 1930s and 1940s in this country. Trends over time in lung cancer death rates, incidence, and survival are presented in greater detail by Devesa in this issue.[4]

A large number of epidemiologic studies have demonstrated the strong association between cigarette smoking and lung cancer in women, as well as men. Large-scale cohort studies that have followed women whose smoking status was known have shown that women who smoke have about a five-fold risk of developing lung cancer compared to nonsmoking women, and that risk increases markedly with amount smoked. There is a clear dose-response relationship of number of cigarettes smoked, years smoked, and type of cigarette to lung cancer risk.[5] Relative risks from studies of males have generally been higher, which is attributed to the fact that, at least in the past, male smokers smoked more cigarettes over more years and were more likely to inhale and to smoke higher tar and nicotine cigarettes and unfiltered cigarettes than were female smokers. Approximately 75% of lung cancer cases in women are attributable to cigarette smoking, making the disease a largely preventable one.[6]

Laryngeal Cancer

Among women who smoke, cancer of the larynx is also substantially increased—fourfold or more compared to nonsmokers, and risk increases with amount of smoking. Risk is particularly elevated among women who both smoke and drink alcohol. The once high ratio of male to female cases of the disease has decreased considerably in recent decades, which is thought to reflect the narrowing of sex differences in smoking (and drinking) prevalence. Although laryngeal cancer is still a relatively uncommon cancer among women, its incidence rates have recently increased markedly.[5]

Esophageal Cancer

Most epidemiologic studies of esophageal cancer have been limited to men, and have consistently demonstrated increased risks of the disease in smokers compared to nonsmokers, as well as what appears to be a strong synergistic effect of cigarette smoking and alcohol use. The 25-state prospective study of the American Cancer Society found that women aged 45-64 who smoked had esophageal cancer mortality rates that were 4.9 times those of nonsmoking women.[7] Risk of esophageal cancer increases dramatically with amount smoked.[5] Incidence rates for the disease in white women have, however, changed only slightly in recent decades;[4] possibly the detrimental effects of smoking have been balanced in the population by other lifestyle changes that are beneficial.

Oral Cavity Cancer

A number of anatomic sites are included in the rubric "oral cavity", including the lip, tongue, mouth, and pharynx, and different epidemiologic studies include varying combinations of these sites. Risk is consistently elevated for smokers across studies, although, again, few studies on women have been reported. American Cancer Society study showed women who smoked to have mortality rates 3.25 times greater than nonsmoking women.[7] As is true for cancers of the larynx and esophagus, there appears to be a strong synergy between smoking and alcohol for oral cavity cancer, such that risk for smokers who drink is much greater than for smokers who do not. Still, smoking appears to be independently related to the disease. Since 1950, rates for oral cancer in women have increased and the male to female ratio of cases has decreased among whites.[5] In the past decade, however, there has been considerable fluctuation in incidence rates.[4]

Bladder Cancer

Various authors have estimated the proportion of female bladder cancers attributable to cigarette smoking in the United States to be around 30 to 40%.[8,9] Smoking appears to increase risk of female bladder cancer two- to threefold, although studies of the dose-response relationship have been less dramatic and somewhat less consistent than for the cancer sites reviewed above.[5] Bladder cancer mortality and incidence rates among white females have been essentially stable since 1950, with the exception of slight increases in incidence rates in the early 1970s.[4,5]

Kidney Cancer

The incidence of kidney cancer has gradually but steadily increased among white women in the U.S. between 1950 and the early 1970s, but has been stable since that time.[4,5] Among whites, the ratio of male to female kidney cancer cases has increased in recent decades, which might not be expected given the narrowing of sex differences in smoking prevalence over time. However, epidemiologic studies have consistently demonstrated an increased risk of kidney cancer among smokers compared to nonsmokers, and the Surgeon General has concluded that cigarette smoking is a contributory factor in the development of the disease.[5]

Pancreatic Cancer

Epidemiologic studies have consistently found a positive association between smoking and pancreatic cancer, with evidence of a dose-response relationship in women as well as men. The relative risk of pancreatic cancer among women who smoked cigarettes compared to nonsmokers in the American Cancer Society 25-state study was 1.4,[7] somewhat lower than has been found in prospective studies of women in other countries.[5] Age-adjusted pancreatic cancer incidence rates in U.S. white women have remained essentially stable since 1950, but the male to female ratio of cases has decreased steadily over the period, and a positive association between mortality rates and smoking patterns in U.S. men and women for the period 1928 to 1978 has been reported.[10] Cigarette smoking is considered by the Surgeon General to be a contributory factor in pancreatic cancer, with perhaps 30% of deaths from the disease due to smoking.[5]

Cervical Cancer

In recent years, a variety of studies in the United States, Canada and Europe have shown a positive association between cigarette smoking and cancer of the uterine cervix. When this relationship was first proposed, it was greeted with skepticism, since it was felt that women who smoke may really be at risk due to early age of first intercourse, multiple sexual partners, or other factors already known to be related to cervical cancer.[11] However, when sexual factors have been controlled in data analysis, smoking still emerges as an independent risk factor, associated with at least a doubling of risk of the disease.[12,13] It is difficult to adequately adjust for sexual and other potential confounders, but evidence for a positive relationship is increasingly more convincing.

The Future of Cigarette Smoking and Cancer in Women

Surveys of smoking prevalence suggest that cigarette smoking reached its peak in the cohort of American women born between 1921 and 1940.[14] However, among women in their early twenties today, smoking prevalence appears to be higher than among women of the same age in past eras.[15] Thus we can expect that—in the absence of major smoking prevention and cessation successes—cancers related to smoking will occupy a major proportion of all female cancers for decades to come.[16] There are some grounds for optimism, however. College-educated women,[17] and girls who are college bound,[18] smoke less than women and girls of lesser education, and so it appears that nonsmoking in women may be "trickling down" the social ladder among women. [In men there has been for some time a clear inverse relation between smoking and social class, whether measured by income or education.[19]] Based on ongoing surveys of high school seniors, it also appears that smoking rates are lower among teenage girls in the 1980s compared to the late 1970s although rates have fluctuated somewhat in very recent years;[18] current national data inclusive of youth who are not in school will be available soon.

Lung cancer rates in women will probably never be as high as the levels experienced by men. Female smoking rates peaked at lower levels than those once attained by men, and a larger proportion of female than male smokers have smoked brands in the lower tar and nicotine categories. Data from several cohort and case-control studies document a lower risk of lung (and other) cancers for smokers of the lower tar and nicotine cigarettes, although their risks are clearly elevated in comparison with those of nonsmokers.[20]

Other Health Effects

Because the concern here is with smoking and cancer, there has been no discussion of the other health-related effects of smoking. Briefly, cigarette smoking is a major contributor to cardiovascular disease in the United States,[21] and the effects of smoking are compounded by use of oral contraceptives. Women who smoke and use the pill increase their risk of myocardial infarction tenfold.[1] Women also experience unique risks related to pregnancy. Smoking increases the risk of miscarriage, stillbirth, low birthweight, and other complications of pregnancy.[1] There are additional concerns related to fire injuries; cigarettes are the leading cause of home fire deaths.

There has been little assessment of the interaction between female smoking and exposures to other carcinogens in the workplace. A wide variety of potential interactions have been described,[22,23] although to date few epidemiologic data on women have been published.

CIGARETTE ADVERTISING AND PROMOTIONS DIRECTED TO WOMEN

Cigarettes have been specifically marketed to women in the United States since the 1920s. Until that time, cigarette smoking was an almost exclusively male behavior. The double standards of the day made smoking socially unacceptable for women, and marketers feared a public backlash should they directly target women in cigarette advertisements. Local ordinances passed in the early part of the century forbade smoking by women in public, and even into the twenties there was much consternation over the issue of female smoking in railroad cars, on campus, and elsewhere. However, during the 1920s social mores and behavior were changing with regard to smoking by women, as reflected in articles on the subject in the lay press. The climate was improving for cigarette manufacturers, and they seized upon the new opportunities during the second half of the decade, with female themes and models featured in the ads; now women were depicted as smokers themselves rather than simply as companions of male smokers [Figure 1]. Change came quickly and by the 1930s cigarette ads were commonplace in popular women's magazines. Themes of sophistication, sexual attractiveness, athleticism, and slimness were already well established in cigarette advertising of the period.[24]

The 1940s was a time of patriotism and cigarette advertising employed related themes. Movie celebrities and other women in uniform were featured, with slogans that capitalized on contributions to the war effort[25] [Figures 2,3]. During the 1950s and 1960s cigarette advertising on radio and television predominated, and advertisements in women's magazines took on a relatively low profile. Near the end of this period, in 1968, Virginia Slims cigarettes were introduced. This was the first brand targeted exclusively to females which achieved great success.[26]

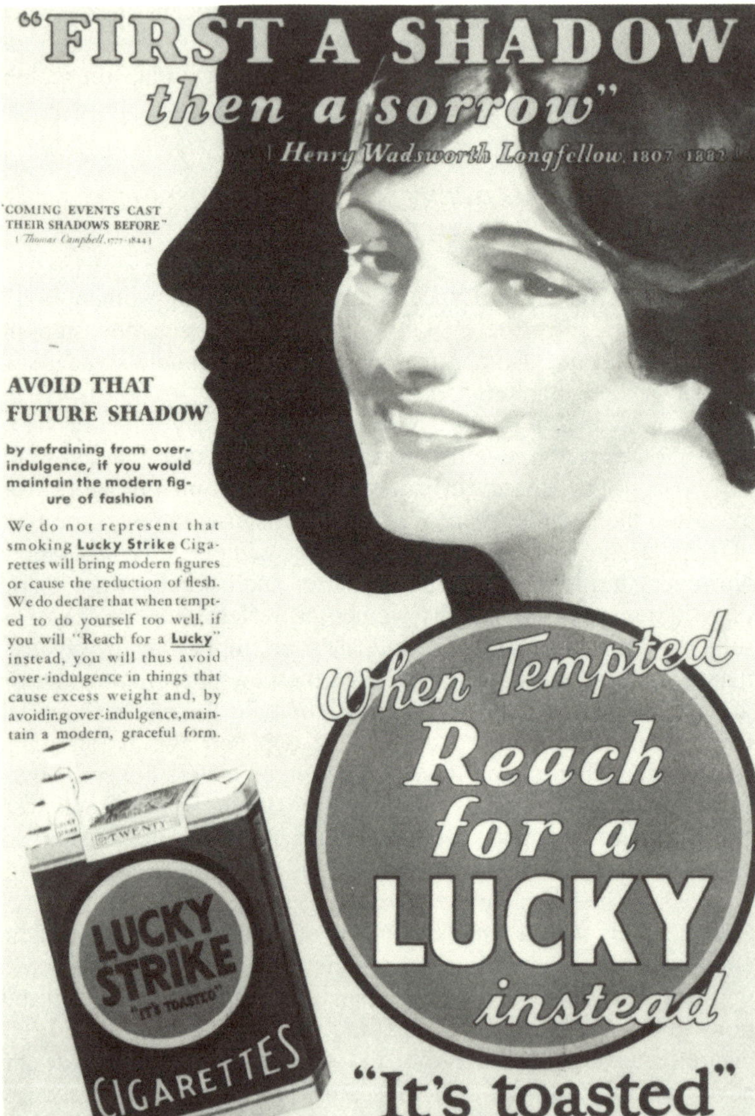

FIGURE 1. "Reach for a Lucky"—from the latter part of the 1920s.

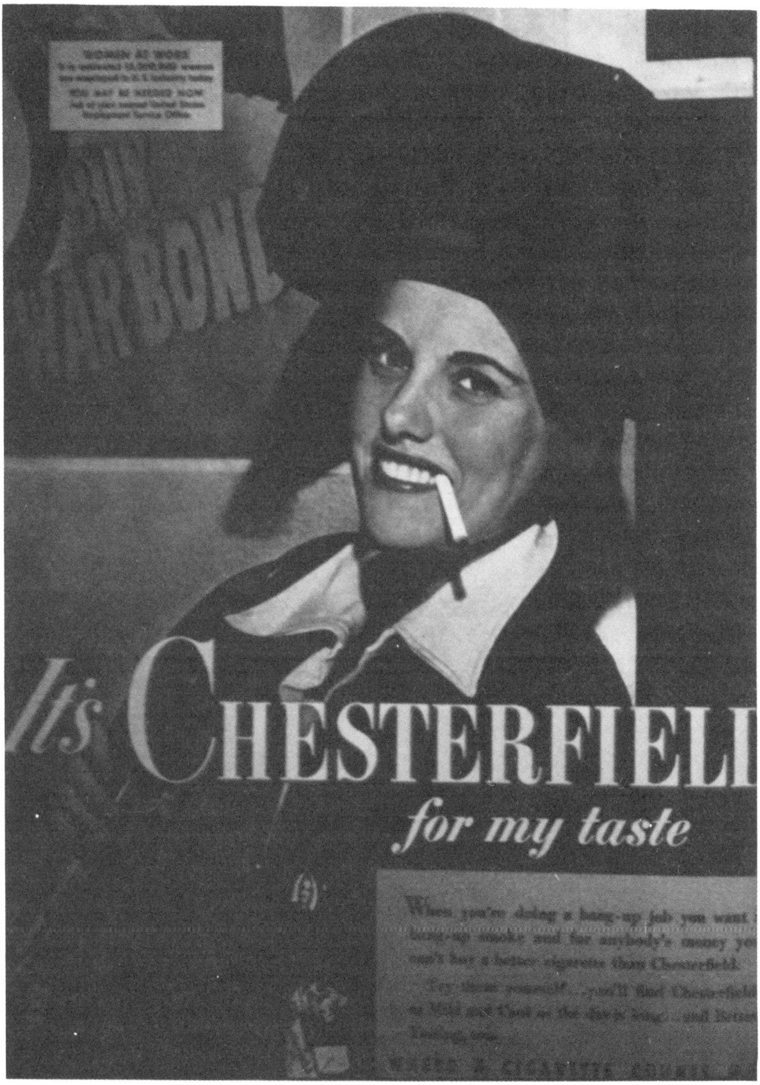

FIGURE 2. "Rosie the Riveter"—from *Better Homes and Gardens*, March 1943, back cover.

On January 2, 1971, the ban on cigarette advertising in the broadcast media went into effect and, contrary to predictions at the time, cigarette advertising in the print media soon began to soar,

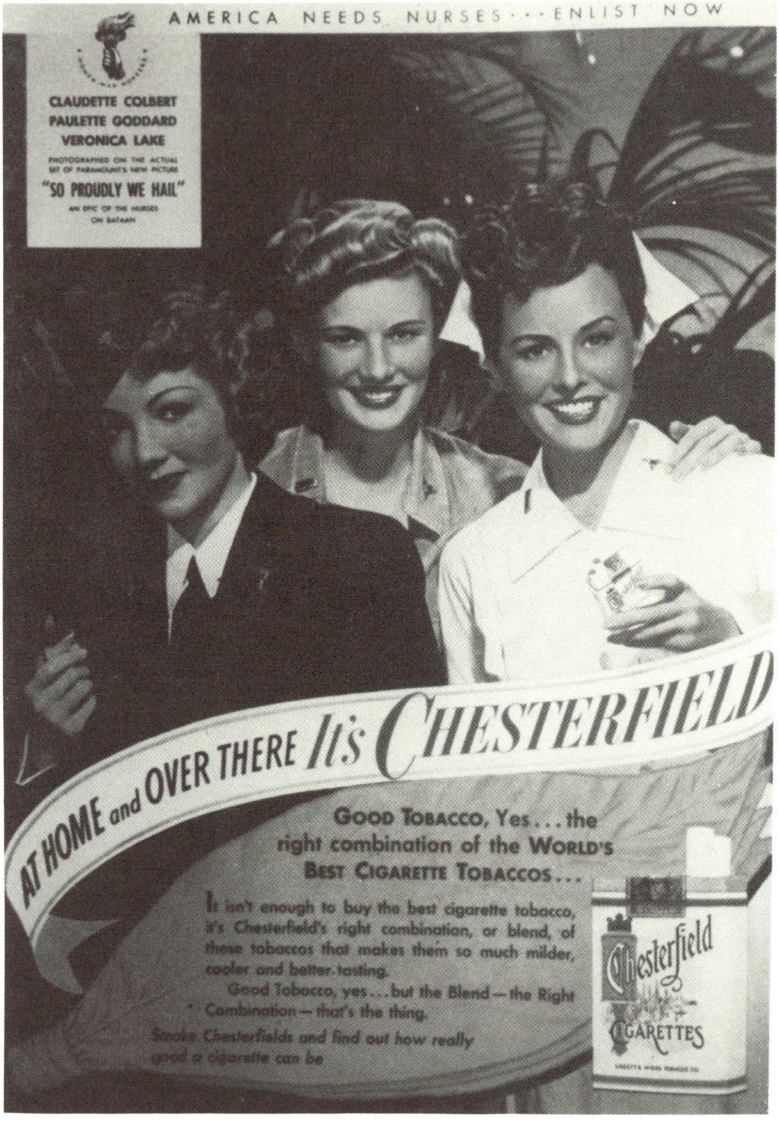
AMERICA NEEDS NURSES . . . ENLIST NOW
CLAUDETTE COLBERT
PAULETTE GODDARD
VERONICA LAKE
PHOTOGRAPHED ON THE ACTUAL SET OF PARAMOUNT'S NEW PICTURE
"SO PROUDLY WE HAIL"
AN EPIC OF THE NURSES ON BATAAN
AT HOME and OVER THERE It's CHESTERFIELD
GOOD TOBACCO, Yes . . . the right combination of the WORLD'S BEST CIGARETTE TOBACCOS . . .
It isn't enough to buy the best cigarette tobacco, it's Chesterfield's right combination, or blend, of these tobaccos that makes them so much milder, cooler and better-tasting.
Good Tobacco, yes . . . but the Blend—the Right Combination—that's the thing.
Smoke Chesterfields and find out how really good a cigarette can be
Chesterfield
CIGARETTES

FIGURE 3. Three celebrities dressed as nurses—from *Better Homes and Gardens*, October 1943, back cover.

quickly outstripping in expenditures the combined print and broadcast advertising budgets of previous years. The women's magazines, which had rarely included even two or three cigarette ads per issue during the 1950s and 1960s, soon experienced an epidemic of cigarette advertising. By the late 1970s, some of the best selling women's magazines included as many as 19 or 20 full pages of cigarette advertising per issue.[24] The notable exception was *Good Housekeeping*, which still maintains its long-standing policy of not accepting cigarette ads.

The 1970s and 1980s have been characterized by the introduction of additional brands marketed specifically to women and by special cigarette promotions for women. Cigarette brands such as Eve, Satin, and Silva Thins joined Virginia Slims in vying for the female market. Other brands, although not marketed exclusively to women, have featured women extensively in their advertising campaigns. The More brand of cigarettes is one example; its advertising features svelte fashion plates with slogans that include "It's long. It's slim. It's elegant. It's More you" [Figure 4]. The recently introduced Ritz brand is the first designer cigarette, with each individual pack and cigarette bearing the "YSL" logo of fashion designer Yves St. Laurent[27] [Figure 5].

Coupons for free or discounted cigarettes are commonly included with ads directed at women, and free cigarette samples are passed out in public places, including distribution of cigarettes at the entrance to tennis matches sponsored by Virginia Slims cigarettes. The sponsorship of professional women's tennis is an obvious example of targeting women and of attempting to link cigarettes with a socially valued activity. [In England, Martina Navratilova appeared at Wimbleton wearing an outfit close in design to the pack of Kim cigarettes, the British counterpart of Virginia Slims cigarettes; until protests were filed, her outfit even bore the Kim logo.[28]] The printed program of the National Organization of Women in the U.S. has been partly underwritten by Philip Morris.[29] In addition, More cigarettes have sponsored a variety of fashion events, including fashion shows in shopping centers throughout the country and awards for designers in the fashion industry.[25,30]

Although not specifically targeted at women, it is of interest that tobacco companies have sponsored such artistic events as the Vatican Art Exhibit (with the Metropolitan Museum of Art), the Joffrey Ballet, the Kool Jazz Festival, the publication of a brochure entitled "Helping Youth Decide" for the National Association of

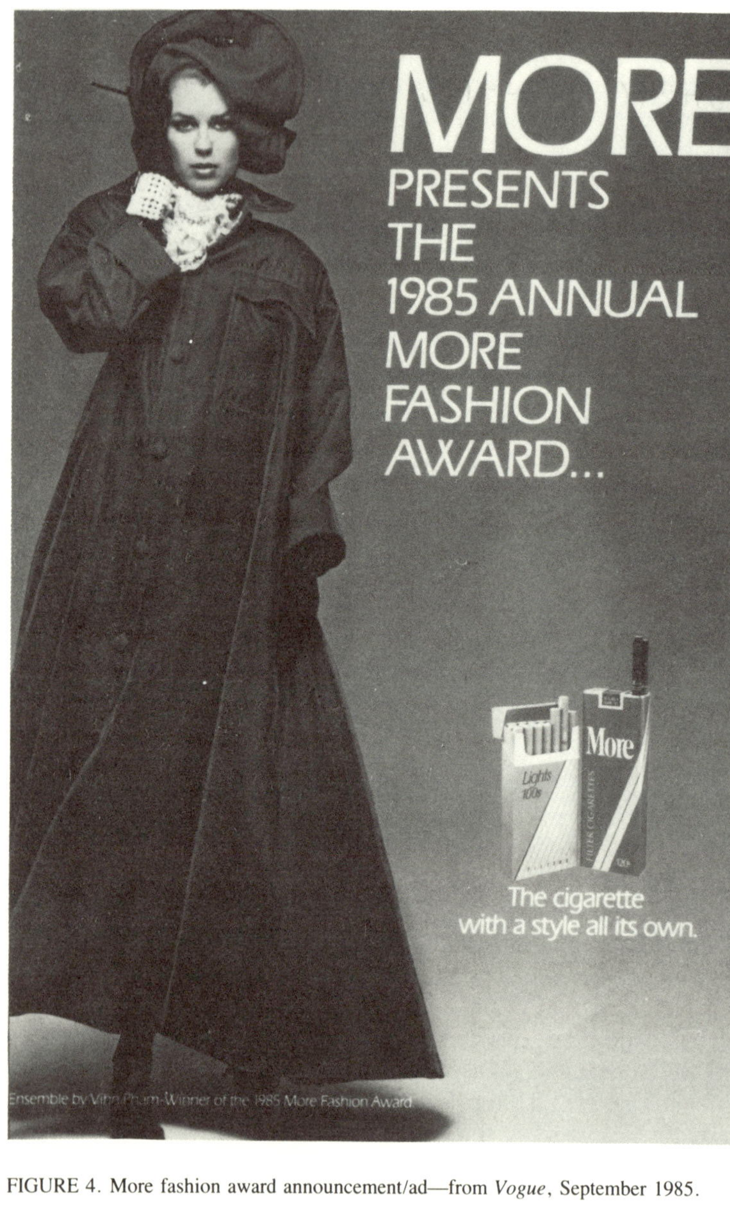

FIGURE 4. More fashion award announcement/ad—from *Vogue*, September 1985.

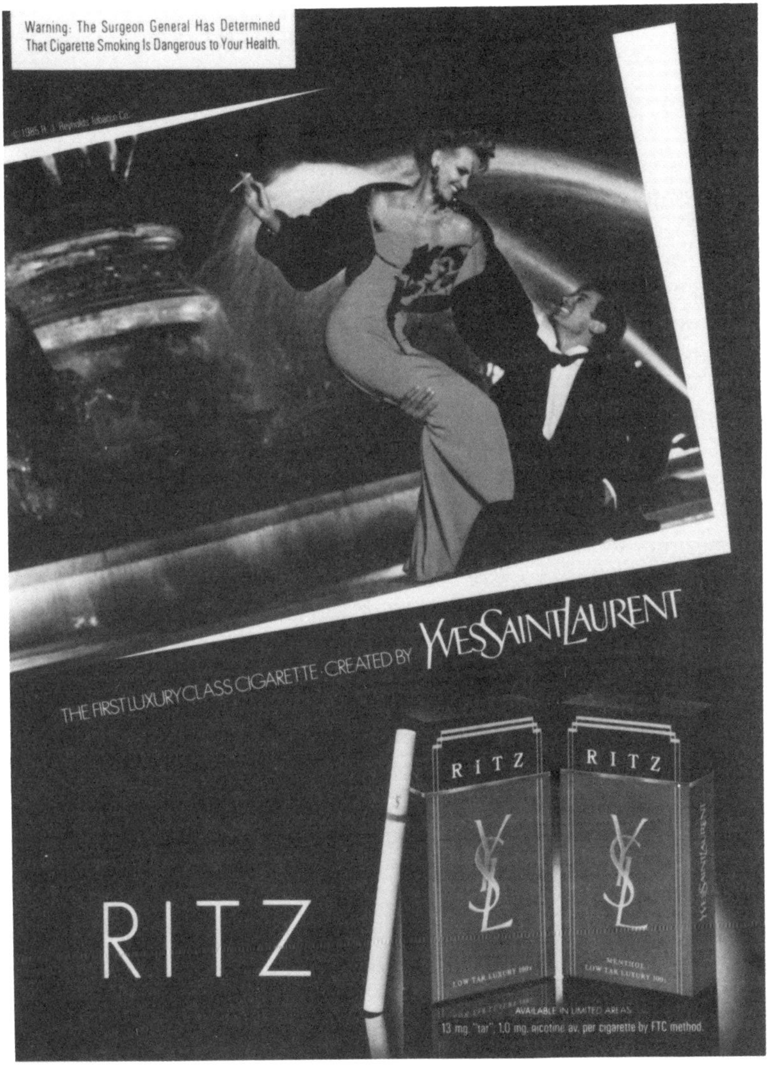

FIGURE 5. Ritz ad—from Washington State regional issue of *Better Homes and Gardens*, July 1985.

State Boards of Education, a golf tournament whose proceeds went to benefit children with cancer, and so on. Such sponsorship can only enhance corporate image and may tend to soften public criticism of tobacco company activities.

EFFORTS TO REDUCE FEMALE SMOKING AND CIGARETTE PROMOTIONS

Activities to Date

The issue of women and smoking is gaining recognition in various ways, including increased attention by the news media.[31–33] In 1982, the first edition of *The Ladykillers: Why Smoking is a Feminist Issue*, written by British author Bobbie Jacobson, was published.[34] The second edition will appear in 1986. Brief pieces in the *New England Journal of Medicine* have called attention to the epidemic of lung cancer in women.[35,36] In 1980, the American Lung Association produced an article entitled "Smoking among women—an equal opportunity tragedy,"[37] and a 1985 editorial in the American Cancer Society's professional journal *CA* was headed, "Lung Cancer: A Feminist Issue."[38] The cover of a 1981 issue of the latter journal featured a beautiful young woman smoking, with a superimposed line plotting the epidemic of lung cancer rates.[39] The American Lung Association and the American Cancer Society have both produced excellent educational materials, posters and public service announcements on women and smoking, including smoking and pregnancy, that are available upon request. In April, 1986, the American Cancer Society held a national conference on cancer control for the leaders of women's organizations around the country, that included presentations on smoking. The National Cancer Institute, through its Divison of Cancer Control and Prevention, has established a women and smoking program through which several intervention projects designed to reduce smoking among women have been funded.

The latest edition of the publication *Our Bodies Ourselves*, produced by the Boston Women's Health Collective, includes several strong references to cigarette smoking. The National Women's Health Network is now actively opposed to women's smoking and is spreading the message through educational activities. The organization participated in a picket of a tennis tournament sponsored by Virginia Slims cigarettes at George Washington University in January of 1985,[40] and held a related press conference at the time of the 1986 tournament in the Washington, D.C. area. Unfortunately, *Ms* magazine[41] and groups representing the women's movement[29] have been noticeably silent on smoking, despite the considerable importance they have attached to other women's health issues. On the other hand, motions to ban smoking during conference sessions have been enthusiastically received at a number of major feminist meetings (Victoria Leonard, National Women's Health Network, personal communication).

Recommended Future Efforts

Many activities can be suggested for those interested in hastening the decline of female smoking and of cigarette promotions targeted to women. Most of the recommendations, of course, apply to men as well.

1. *Encourage smoking prevention programs for pre-teens and early teens in the schools.* Cigarette smoking in the U.S. today is a habit that is usually regularly established by the age of 16.[1] Rarely does smoking initiation begin in adulthood. Most experimentation with cigarettes occurs in the early teen years. Thus, to be effective, prevention programs must begin early. It is generally felt that simply reciting the long-term health effects has little impact on young people, for whom those consequences are too remote in time. Rather, effective programs should incorporate information about the undesirable short-term effects (smoker's breath, yellow fingernails, foul-smelling clothes, loss of spending money), help students to recognize the deceptiveness and manipulativeness of cigarette advertising, and bring them to understand that cigarette smoking is addictive and, therefore, leads to loss of control.

2. *Be supportive of smokers who wish to quit and prepared to inform them about smoking cessation programs.* Numerous studies show that smoking cessation greatly reduces risk of cancer and other diseases. Most smokers wish they could quit and a large proportion have attempted to quit already. Tens of millions of Americans are ex-smokers and the vast majority have quit on their own, outside of a formal smoking cessation program. Most people who have successfully quit report having attempted more than once to do so; thus failure to quit the first time should not be a deterrent to trying again. A variety of techniques have been recommended in formal programs that may work for individuals, including adoption of substitute behaviors (chewing gum or ice cubes, occupying one's hands with beads or needlework), exercise, careful attention to diet (so as to not gain weight, become discouraged, and relapse), avoidance of situations that tempt one to smoke, and a reward system (such as treating oneself with the money saved from not purchasing cigarettes). Some

people keep diaries of their smoking patterns before quitting to be familiar with the context of their smoking and learn how best to deal with their own situation. Among the many formal smoking cessation programs available are the "Fresh Start" programs offered by the American Cancer Society and the "Freedom from Smoking" offered by the American Lung Association. Information can be obtained by calling the local chapters of these organizations.

It has been suggested that women have more difficulty with smoking cessation than men, but current evidence for this view is not strong [see review of the subject by Orlandi in this issue[42]]. Special programs have been developed for women, particularly pregnant women. Programs targeted to pregnant women are important for several reasons. Because of the risks to fetal health, pregnant smokers are highly motivated to quit. Moreover, since most women become pregnant and most do so at relatively young ages, there is great potential for reaching a sizeable proportion of female smokers and interrupting their smoking careers early in life through such programs. Support from friends and loved ones, smokers and nonsmokers alike, should help to increase the likelihood of quitting.

3. *Support nonsmoking legislation and policies in public places, at work, and in the home.* It is easy to support a nonsmoking society by placing tasteful nonsmoking signs in the home and workplace and by making it clear to friends and associates that smoke-free air is one's preference. Institutional policies or legislated ordinances that prohibit smoking in public places take the burden off the individual and help to insure a smoke-free environment for all. Writing letters to legislators on behalf of proposed legislation or actually initiating such legislation at the local level is to be strongly encouraged. Organizations supporting such activities are Americans for Nonsmokers Rights, headquartered in Berkeley, California, and ASH (Action on Smoking and Health), based in Washington, D.C.

4. *Write to the editors and publishers of women's magazines to let them know your concerns about their acceptance of cigarette advertising.* It is dismaying that cigarette advertising increased dramatically in the 1970s despite the then well-known medical evidence regarding the serious health consequences for women. Inclusion of cigarette ads in women's magazines suggests to the reader than these publications condone cigarette smoking. Of perhaps greater concern is the mounting evidence that editorial coverage of smoking and health issues in popular magazines has been restrained or even cen-

sored, out of fear of offending tobacco advertisers.[43–45] Given that women's magazines are a major source of health-related information for many women, such editorial restraint could result in serious misperceptions of risk on the part of the public. Consumers might seriously consider cancelling subscriptions to magazines that accept cigarette advertising, with a note to the publisher clearly stating why. It has been recommended that physicians put bold slashes across cigarette ads in all the magazines they have in their office waiting rooms or cancel subscriptions to magazines that carry such ads, as one way of sending a clear health education message to patients.[46] Parents can take similar opportunities at home, helping their children to recognize the discordance between the positive images in the cigarette ads and the reality of what really happens to so many people who smoke.

5. *Protest cigarette company sponsorship of sporting and fashion events, of the arts, and of educational and medical programs.* Such sponsorship is only possible because of cigarette profits that have come at the expense of hundreds of thousands of cancer and other smoking-related deaths. Individual women and women's groups can let the organizers of such events know of their strong objections to linking cigarettes with socially valued activities. Informational pickets can be held at the entrance to such events, with press releases issued in advance, as was done by a San Francisco women's group at the time of the Virginia Slims tennis finals in the San Francisco Bay Area, January 1984. Women in leadership positions, especially the members of boards of directors of artistic and other institutions, should be committed to resist the temptation of accepting such sponsorship. Female celebrities—tennis stars, fashion models, ballerinas, and musicians—should speak out against the association of cigarettes with their professional endeavors.

6. *Encourage women's groups to see smoking as a feminist issue, to refuse cigarette sponsorship of their events, and to increase public awareness of attempts by the industry to associate itself with women's activities.* The newsletters and newspapers of women's groups can publicize the myriad health risks faced by women who smoke, putting smoking in perspective with other health concerns women face, and can increase public awareness of attempts by the industry to be seen as an ally of women. The leaders of women's organizations can take public stands decrying tobacco industry promotions in the face of the epidemic of female lung cancer. Discussion of smoking-related topics should be included in the

programs of women's conferences. Obviously women's organizations have many other social, political, and health issues on their agendas. But, given that in 1986 an estimated 41,100 American women will die of lung cancer,[47] not to mention other smoking-related diseases, it is paramount that smoking be seen as a feminist priority.

NOTES

1. Office on Smoking and Health. (1980). The Health Consequences of Smoking for Women. A Report of the Surgeon General. Rockville, MD: Public Health Service, U.S. Department of Health and Human Services.

2. Loeb, L.A., Ernster, V.L., Warner, K.E., Abbotts, J., & Laszlo, J. (1984). Smoking and lung cancer: An overview. *Cancer Res* 44:5940–5958.

3. Silverberg, E. (1985). Cancer statistics, 1985. *CA* 35:19–35.

4. Devesa, S.S. (1986). Cancer mortality, incidence, and patient survival among American Women. *Women and Health* 11:7–22.

5. Office on Smoking and Health. (1982). The Health Consequences of Smoking. Cancer. A Report of the Surgeon General. Rockville, MD: Public Health Service, U.S. Department of Health and Human Services.

6. Doll, R., & Peto, R. (1981). The Causes of Cancer: Quantitative Estimates of Avoidable Risks of Cancer in the United States Today. Oxford: Oxford University Press.

7. Hammond, E.C., & Seidman, H. (1980). Smoking and cancer in the United States. *Prev Med* 9:169–173.

8. Wynder, E.L., & Goldsmith, R. (1977). The epidemiology of bladder cancer. A second look. *Cancer 40*:1246–1268.

9. Cole, P., Monson, R.R., Haning, H., & Friedell, G.H. (1971). Smoking and cancer of the lower urinary tract. *N. Engl. J. Med.* 284:129–134.

10. Weiss, W., & Benarde, M.A. (1983). The temporal relation between cigarette smoking and pancreatic cancer. *Am J Public Health* 73: 1403–1404.

11. Stellman, S.D., Austin, H., & Wynder, E.L. (1980). Cervix cancer and cigarette smoking: A case-control study. *Am J Epidemiol* 111:383–388.

12. Lyon, J.L., Gardner, J.W., West, D.W., Stanish, W.M., & Hebertson RM. (1983). Smoking and carcinoma *in situ* of the uterine cervix. *Am J Public Health* 73:558–562.

13. Trevathan,E.,Layde,P.,Webster,L.A.,Adams,J.B.,Benigno,B.B.,&Ory,H.(1983). Cigarette smoking and dysplasia and carcinoma of the uterine cervix. *JAMA* 250:499–502.

14. Harris, J.E. (1983). Cigarette smoking among successive birth cohorts of men and women in the United States during 1900–80. *JNCI* 71:473–479.

15. Remington, P.L., Forman, M.R., Gentry, E.M., Marks, J.S., Hogelin, G.C., Trowbridge, F.L. (1985). Current smoking trends in the United States. *JAMA* 253:2975–2978.

16. Cummings, K.M. (1984). Changes in the smoking habits of adults in the United States and recent trends in lung cancer mortality. *Cancer Detect Prev* 7:125–134.

17. Office on Smoking and Health. (1979). Smoking and Health. A Report of the Surgeon General. Rockville, MD: Public Health Service, U.S. Department of Health, Education and Welfare.

18. Johnston, L.D., Bachman, J.G., & O'Malley, P.M. (1982). Student Drug Use, Attitudes, and Beliefs: National Trends, 1975–1982. Rockville, MD: U.S. Department of Health and Human Services, Public Health Service, National Institute on Drug Abuse.

19. Wynder, E.L., & Stellman, S.D. (1977). Comparative epidemiology of tobacco-related cancers. *Cancer Res* 37:4608–4622.

20. Stellman, S.D. (1986). Cigarette yield and cancer risk: Evidence from case-control and prospective studies. *In* Zaridze, D., Peto, R., (Eds.). *Tobacco: A Major International Health Hazard (IARC Scientific Publication No. 74).* Lyon, International Agency for Research on Cancer.

21. Office on Smoking and Health. (1983). The Health Consequences of Smoking: Cardiovascular Disease. A Report of the Surgeon General. Rockville, MD: Public Health Service, U.S. Department of Health and Human Services.

22. Stellman, S.D., & Stellman, J.M. (1981). Women's occupations, smoking, and cancer and other diseases. *CA* 31:29–43.

23. Office on Smoking and Health. (1985). The health consequences of smoking: Cancer and chronic lung disease in the workplace. A report of the Surgeon General. Rockville, MD: Public Health Service, U.S. Department of Health and Human Services.

24. Ernster, V.L. (1985). Mixed messages for women: A social history of cigarette smoking and advertising. *NY State J Med* 85:335–340.

25. Ernster, V.L. (in press). Advertising and marketing of cigarettes to women. Chapter in: M.J. Rosenberg (ed.). *Smoking and Reproductive Health.* Boston: PSG.

26. Robinson, W.A. (1985, May 30). Virginia Slims come a long way in 17 years. *Advertising Age*, p. 30.

27. Gloede, W.F. (1985, January 21). RJR puts on the Ritz. *Advertising Age*, pp. 1,78.

28. Navratilova's outfit angers non-smokers. (1983, June 27). *The Guardian.*

29. Shear, M. (1985). The pro-death lobby. *The Women's Review of Books* 2:6–8.

30. More fashion award dinner. (1985, May 30–June 19). U.S. Tobacco and Candy Journal.

31. Brody, J.E. (1985, January 16). Lung cancer is expected to become a top killer of women. *New York Times.*

32. Okie, S. (1985, November 11). Smoking now worst threat to women's health. *Washington Post*, pp. A1, A16.

33. Seligman, J. (1985, November 25). Women smokers: The risk factor. *Newsweek*, pp. 76–78.

34. Jacobson, B. (1982). *The Ladykillers: Why Smoking is a Feminist Issue*. New York: Continuum.

35. Starzyk, P.M. (1983). Lung-cancer deaths: Equality by 2000? *N Engl J Med* 308: 1289.

36. Stolley, P.D. (1983). Lung cancer in women—five years later, situation worse. *N Engl J Med* 308:428–429.

37. Doyle, N.C. (1980, July/August). Smoking among women—an equal opportunity tragedy. American Lung Association Bulletin.

38. Holleb, A.I. (1985). Lung cancer: A feminist issue. *CA* 35:125–126.

39. Holleb, A.I. (1981). Smoking: The ticking time bomb for teenage girls. *CA* 31:44–45.

40. Hogue, C.J.R., & Berman, S.M. (in press). Smoking and the women's movement. Chapter in: M.J. Rosenberg (ed.). *Smoking and Reproductive Health.* Boston: PSG.

41. Cromer, M.A. (1983). "Precious baby." *NY State J Med* 83:1292–1293.

42. Orlandi, M.A. (1986). Gender differences in smoking cessation. *Women and Health* 11:237–251.

43. Smith, R.C. (1978). The magazines' smoking habit. *Columbia Journalism Review* 16:29–31.

44. Whelan, E.M., Sheridan, M.J., Meister, K.A., & Mosher, B.A. (1981). Analysis of coverage of tobacco hazards in women's magazines. *J Public Health Policy* 2:28–35.

45. Warner, K.E. (1985). Cigarette advertising and media coverage of smoking and health. *N Engl J Med* 312:384–388.

46. Richards, J.W. (1983) A positive health strategy for the office waiting room. *NY State J Med* 83:1358–1360.

47. American Cancer Society. (1986). *Facts and Figures, 1986.* American Cancer Society, New York.

Gender Differences in Smoking Cessation

Mario A. Orlandi, PhD, MPH

ABSTRACT. Men and women have traditionally consumed cigarettes very differently, demonstrating widely varying patterns of prevalence during the past eight decades. For example, though the prevalance of smoking among men increased dramatically soon after the turn of the century, an analogous though less dramatic increase among women was not observed for another 25–30 years. Similarly, when a dramatic decrease in smoking prevalence among men was observed following the 1964 Surgeon General's Report, a comparable decrease among women was not seen until 15 years later. Such differences in smoking patterns have led to the widespread belief that giving up smoking is more difficult for women than it is for men. This paper reviews various studies which address this issue and suggests areas in which further research is needed.

INTRODUCTION

Historically, women and men in the United States have differed considerably with respect to their use of cigarettes (Howe, 1984). The dramatic increase in cigarette consumption observed soon after 1900 which continued throughout the next five decades was due primarily to smoking in males (USDHHS, 1979). In the early 1900s strong social pressure inhibited smoking among women and it was not until the 1920s that women were even depicted in cigarette advertising (Tenant, 1950). Although the available data from the early 1900s is somewhat unclear, the best estimates suggest that the growth of smoking among women occurred much more gradually and lagged behind the increases observed in males by at least 25-30 years (USDHHS, 1979). Throughout the 1940s women's smoking rates continued to accelerate and in the 1950s this acceleration was

Mario A. Orlandi is Chief, Division of Health Promotion Research, American Health Foundation, 320 E. 43rd St., New York, NY 10017. Supported in part by National Cancer Institutes Grants CA38219 and CA41621.

fueled by the introduction of the filtertip cigarette. Per capita consumption of cigarettes reached a peak in 1963. In the early 1960s prevalence of regular cigarette smoking had reached 52 percent among males and 33 percent among females (USDHEW, 1970).

Since the 1960s, however, cigarette smoking prevalence has generally declined. Following the appearance in January 1964 of the first report of the Advisory Committee to the Surgeon General (USDHEW, 1964), the prevalence of regular cigarette use among males has steadily declined. From 1965 to 1978, the prevalence of adult male cigarette smokers declined from 51 to 37 percent. During this time period, however, a comparable decline among female smokers was not observed. From 1965 to 1976, smoking prevalence among females remained virtually unchanged, though since 1976 the proportion of women smokers has gradually declined to below 30 percent (USDHEW, 1979). Just as with the onset of widespread cigarette use prior to 1965, the national trend toward a decline in cigarette consumption since 1965 has occurred more gradually in females and has lagged behind the trend observed in males by a number of years.

While a number of factors are known to have contributed to the changes in smoking prevalence described above, changes in smoking cessation rates are believed to have played a particularly significant role (Harris, 1979). Since gender differences with regard to smoking prevalence have been consistently dramatic and since smoking cessation has been identified as a key factor in explaining the overall decline in prevalence since 1965, the question has been raised repeatedly as to whether or not women have greater difficulty giving up smoking than men do (USDHHS, 1979; Jarvis, 1984). This paper will address this highly complex question in three ways: first, by identifying the major issues and hypotheses that are relevant to the study of sex differences in smoking cessation; second, by critically reviewing the available literature on this topic; and third, by pointing out several significant gaps in our understanding of this issue and areas in which future research is needed.

ISSUES AND HYPOTHESES

The 1979 Surgeon General's Report on the health consequences of smoking for women states unequivocally that, across all reported smoking cessation treatment studies "women have more difficulty giving up smoking than men, both at the end of treatment and at long-term points of measurement'' (USDHHS, 1979, p. 307). A claim such as this, if supported, carries very different implications for our general approach to cancer control among women than does the claim that men and women differ with respect to smoking prevalence and rates of cessation. If women actually experience *greater difficulty* than men do in giving up smoking, then smoking cessation intervention approaches should attempt to take this into account. In order to critically evaluate the data which may or may not support this contention, it is necessary to first identify the various categories of relevant variables that could be used to measure sex differences in smoking cessation. For the purposes of this paper these variable categories will also serve as a framework for identifying gaps in our current knowledge and areas in which further research is needed.

Cigarette smoking is a learned behavior that induces over time both physiological and psychological dependence in participants. Smoking cessation is a process which involves relearning and the breakdown of established response patterns. This type of behavior change, or lifestyle reorientation, has been studied extensively because of its implications for public health promotion. Several categories of variables have been identified through this research that are known to be factors in the success or failure of efforts to alter lifestyle habits. These include: *predisposing factors* (either physiological or psychological factors already existing prior to the attempt to alter one's behavior which can potentially affect results); *enabling factors* (any environmental or sociocultural factors that act to facilitate or inhibit the attempt to alter one's behavior) and *reinforcing factors* (the perceived and expected positive and negative consequences associated with the attempt to alter one's behavior). For each category of variable that can be identified, a hypothesis can be generated regarding potentially relevant sex differences. A representative list of such predisposing, reinforcing, and enabling factors and their related hypotheses follows:

Predisposing Variables and Related Hypotheses

V1: physiological or metabolic factors

H1: There are physiological or metabolic differences between men and women which influence the way in which cessation, withdrawal, and long-term maintainance are experienced.

V2: degree of difficulty in quitting

H2: Due to a variety of factors, it is inherently more difficult (i.e., requires a greater effort) for women to give up smoking than for men.

V3: tolerance for discomfort related to quitting

H3: Though it requires an equal amount of effort, women are less able than men to tolerate the discomforts related to cessation, withdrawal, and long-term maintainence.

Enabling Variables and Related Hypotheses

V4: organized intervention availability

H4: Organized interventions are more available to men than they are to women.

V5: utilization of available organized interventions

H5: More men than women avail themselves of organized cessation interventions (clinics, books, television programs, etc.)

V6: organized intervention effectiveness

H6: Organized interventions are more effective for men than they are for women.

Reinforcing Variables and Related Hypotheses

V7: psychosocial contingencies

H7: The psychosocial factors which influence cigarette smoking, both positively and negatively, are categorically different for women than for men.

V8: psychosocial contingency weighting.

H8: Though contingencies are not categorically different, women weight these contingencies differently than men do and therefore consider some more salient than others.

Similarly, the behavioral factors relevant to the study of gender differences in smoking cessation can be analyzed in terms of specific hypotheses. A representative list of these variables follows:

Behavioral Variables and Related Hypotheses

V9: cessation attempt rates

H9: A higher percentage of men than women who smoke try to quit.

V10: cessation success rates
H10: A higher percentage of men than women who attempt to quit are successful.
V11: long-term maintainance rates
H11: A higher percentage of men than women who do quit are still abstinent after 6 months.

Though far from exhaustive, these lists of variables and related hypotheses provides an overview of the types of factors that are likely to be responsible for gender differences in smoking cessation if such differences were found to be significant. While relatively little research has been carried out on this specific topic, a number of relevant studies have been conducted and will be described here. As will be obvious from the review which follows, much of the pertinent data that would be required to answer the questions posed by this paper are not available.

OVERVIEW OF RELEVANT RESEARCH

Data Related to Predisposing Factors

The variables described above as V1, V2, and V3 are examples of factors that could potentially predispose women, differentially, to lower smoking quit rates and success rates than men. For example, a measurable and consistent difference in the metabolism of nicotine could provide a rationale for sex differences in smoking cessation. While several studies have suggested possible differences in the way that men and women metabolize nicotine (Garrod and Jenner, 1975) no clear cut differences have yet to be demonstrated, and most of the observed differences were most probably caused by variations in inhalation depth and other topographical smoking patterns (Schievelbein et al., 1978). Furthermore, physiological differences are likely to be unrelated to the improved cessation rates observed in adult women since 1979.

A number of studies have reported other sex-linked factors, however, that have been described as inherent mechanisms that could predispose women to greater difficulty in smoking cessation. For example, it has been reported that women experience stress in their daily lives that is both qualitatively and quantitatively different from that experienced by men (Burns, 1969). Since stress has been causally linked to both cessation difficulty and relapse (Shiffman,

1979; Lichtenstein et al., 1977) this may be a predisposing factor that contributes to smoking cessation differences in men and women. Other studies have supported this relationship. For example, Cherry and Kiernan (1976) found that women who smoke have higher scores on personality scales which measure neuroticism, and that this tendency is observable in women prior to becoming a smoker as well. Burns (1969) also reported this finding and showed, furthermore, that analogous differences were not found in men. Similarly, a survey of young women and teenage girls conducted by Yankelovich et al. (1977) reported that women smokers were characterized by apprehension and tension, factors which these respondents also linked to an inability to give up smoking. Various other studies have also compared men and women with regard to psychological distress and difficulty experienced in quitting smoking. Russell (1970), for example, reported that dropping out of treatment for reasons related to depression was more frequent, and the reported symptoms more severe, among women. Similarly, Peterson et al. (1968) reported that 43 percent of women in their sample described nervousness as the primary reason for resuming smoking after quitting, whereas only 23 percent of men reported this.

The severity of symptoms experienced during withdrawal are known to be related to the likelihood of relapse, especially during the initial period following cessation (Guilford, 1967). In an analysis of previously published data, Shiffman (1979) demonstrated that the majority of symptoms reported by subjects to be related to relapse were more frequently reported by women than by men. Other studies have not, however, reported significant gender differences in the perceived severity of withdrawal symptoms (Trahair, 1967; Peterson et al., 1968), which has left this issue open to question.

Data Related to Enabling Factors

One type of enabling factor known to influence smoking cessation is the availability and utilization of known behavior change techniques. A great deal of research has been devoted to the study of smoking cessation techniques in an effort to determine which of these, either alone or in combination, are the most effective (Lichtenstein & Brown, 1980). This research, however, was not designed to look specifically at gender differences, and a relatively small percentage of the studies that have been reported even provide a breakdown of results by sex. Nonetheless, a recent review evaluated 39 studies of smoking cessation effectiveness in which gender differences could be evaluated (USDHHS, 1979). These studies fell into five categories: skills training and education, physician advice, pharmacotherapy, psychotherapy, and behavior modification. Across all treatment categories, women were reported to have lower end of treatment success rates than men. In none of these 39 studies were women significantly more successful than men.

The interventions described in this review were not attended more frequently by men. The majority, in fact reported higher participation rates for women, suggesting that utilization patterns and availability are not factors that would explain the apparent gender differences in reported success rates.

Data Related to Reinforcing Factors

A substantial body of research has suggested that women and men have traditionally smoked cigarettes for different reasons. Both the positive reinforcements promoting smoking and the negative reinforcements inhibiting quitting have been reported to be different. Several studies, for example, have suggested women are more likely than men to smoke in order to reduce unpleasant feelings (Ikard & Tomkins, 1973). Similarly, nationwide surveys have supported the contention that more women are "negative affect" smokers than men and that there is no difference between men and women with regard to "positive affect" smoking (USDHEW, 1969; USDHEW, 1973). Cigarettes have also been described by women as a method for breaking up time periods during the day, for promoting physical autonomy from children, and for providing role differentiation (Graham, 1976), considerations which are infrequently, if ever, given by men as reasons for smoking. Another study which reported gender differences in treatment success rates noted that unsuccessful women, as opposed to men, described cigarettes as "companions" and cited the difficulty of being deprived of outside activities and adult companionship during the day as primary barriers to quitting (Wilhelmsen, 1968). This study suggested further that the lower cessation rates of women were due almost entirely to the unsuccessful attempts of homemakers to quit smoking.

Another significant reinforcing factor which is believed to influence the success of smokers who attempt to quit is the tendency to engage in symptom substitution following cessation and the perceived negative consequences of this tendency (Bozzetti, 1972). In particular, women smokers are reported to be more concerned than men that they will gain weight if they quit (USDHEW, 1976).

Data Related to Behavioral Factors

The behavioral variables listed above (V9, V10, and V11) are examples of data related to smoking prevalence and smoking cessation that has been collected through a variety of national surveys over the past several decades. A review of the available survey data of this type is necessary in order to determine if and when reliable gender differences have been reported relative to smoking cessation patterns.

Various authors have traced the evolution of cigarette smoking among successive generations of American women and men during the twentieth century (Tennant, 1950; USDCBC, 1975; Jackson, 1950; Hammond & Garfinkel, 1968). In general, throughout this period, women have differed from men in smoking prevalence and the rate of diffusion of the smoking habit both within and between birth cohorts. While smoking among men increased rapidly during the years before and during World War I, the widespread onset of smoking among women did not begin until 25–30 years later (USDHHS, 1979). After 1940, smoking rates among women increased rapidly as more women entered the urban labor force. During the 1940s and the 1950s men continued to smoke at higher rates than women, but women continued to close the gap (Haenszel et al., 1956). In 1949, the Gallup Poll reported that 54 percent of adult males and 33 percent of adult females were smokers (American Institute of Public Opinion, 1977). Per capita consumption of cigarettes reached a peak in 1963 which has not been observed since (USDHEW, 1964). A decline in consumption began to occur immediately following the appearance in January 1964 of the First Report of the Advisory Committee to the Surgeon General on Smoking and Health (USDHEW, 1964). It is the period following 1964 that is most important for the topic which this paper addresses, since it is at this point in the history of cigarette use that smoking prevalence began to dramatically decline and relevant differences between men and women with respect to cessation rates began to emerge.

Among adult males, cigarette smoking prevalence has declined continuously since the 1964 Surgeon General's Report. Between the years 1970 and 1979, three indicators were used to track the contribution of smoking cessation to the overall decrease in smoking prevalence: (1) the percent of all recent smokers who made a "fairly serious attempt to quit" within the previous twelve months; (2) the percent of smokers attempting to quit who reported their attempt a success; and (3) the percent of recent smokers who reported successful quitting within the previous twelve months.

As Table One indicates, all three indicators were significantly higher in 1970 for men than for women. Fewer women, proportionally, than men attempted to quit in that year, and for those who made the attempt, their probability of success was significantly lower. While self-reported measures of this type are known to suffer from various limitations, these data are considered the best estimates available of overall annual cessation rates.

While quit attempt rates have declined in general since 1970,

TABLE ONE: Estimated rates of attempted and successful cessation among adult recent cigarette smokers; United States, 1970–1979.

	(1)	(2)	(3)
WOMEN			
1970	40.8	21.3	8.7
1975	30.2	19.5	5.9
1978	32.7	18.8	6.2
1979	32.9	21.6	7.0
MEN			
1970	44.4	26.4	11.7
1975	28.3	20.1	5.7
1978	29.1	21.5	6.3
1979	31.4	21.3	6.7

(1) Percent of recent smokers who attempted to quit during the past year.

(2) Percent of smokers attempting to quit during past year who reported success.

(3) Percent of all recent smokers who reported successfully quitting during past year.

SOURCE: USDHEW (1973, 1975, 1979).

both the probability of attempting to quit and the probability of success were by 1979 virtually equivalent for adult men and women and these trends have continued since that time (USDHHS, 1983). By 1979, approximately one in three adult smokers (men and women) were making a serious attempt to quit during the course of a year and approximately one in five of those who attempted to quit were successful (USDHHS, 1979). Similarly, it has been observed that, with each successive birth cohort, women have become increasingly similar to men in terms of other smoking-related variables such as daily cigarette consumption and types of cigarettes consumed (USDHHS, 1982).

Table Two shows the length of time off cigarettes for current smokers following their most recent attempt to quit. A smaller proportion of the total smoking population relapsed within 6 months, 1 year, or 2-1/2 years in 1980 as compared to 1966. In 1966, 80.1% of quitters resumed smoking within 6 months, whereas by 1980 this proportion had decreased to 72.2%. This reduction in the percentage of relapse was reported for both men and women. In general a higher percentage of male current smokers than female current smokers reported that their attempt to quit lasted more than six months—in both 1975 and 1980. Despite this trend, the data do not, however, suggest a significant difference in relapse rate by gender. By 2-1/2 years, in fact, the rates for males and females of all ages over 21 are essentially equal. It is important to note that the gender differences which do persist at 2-1/2 years are accounted for primarily by the 21-24 year old females who report a 100% relapse rate by 2-1/2 years.

SUMMARY AND DISCUSSION

To summarize, behavioral self-report data have supported the hypothesis that women have historically been less successful than men at giving up smoking. This was particularly true during the years following the 1965 Surgeon General's Report. Since 1979, however, smoking cessation trends among adult women have become increasingly similar to those observed in men. The only subgroup of the female population that has not yet demonstrated smoking decreases comparable to males is the adolescent female population. The lack of a more marked decline overall in the proportion of cigarette smokers among women can be explained primarily by the increase

TABLE TWO: Cumulative percentage of relapse of current cigarette smokers during their last attempt to quit smoking; United States, 1966, 1975, and 1980.

Gender, age and education	1966[1] <6 mo	1966[1] <1 yr	1966[1] <2½ yr	1975[1] <6mo	1975[1] <1 yr	1975[1] <2½ yr	1980[2] <6mo	1980[2] <1 yr	1980[2] <2½ yr
All who attempted	80.1	89.5	96.6	71.3	83.1	94.3	72.2	84.3	94.9
Males									
All ages 21	79.5	88.7	96.3	69.0	82.2	94.0	67.9	81.2	93.6
21-24	93.6	100.0	-	77.4	91.1	100.0	76.5	91.9	97.1
25-34	79.4	90.0	98.5	70.6	84.5	96.4	67.1	80.3	96.6
35-44	75.7	87.8	95.3	64.3	77.6	93.1	61.7	75.9	90.7
45-54	80.8	84.2	95.2	69.3	82.0	92.2	65.6	76.6	91.4
55-64	73.7	86.9	93.5	71.7	80.7	92.8	72.0	84.7	91.3
≥65	78.2	84.5	93.9	59.7	77.5	85.3	71.1	86.1	94.3
Female									
All ages 21	80.3	90.3	96.6	75.4	84.4	94.9	77.0	87,8	96.2
21-24	80.2	97,3	99.9	83.4	91.7	97.4	85.4	95.6	100.0
25-34	81.9	92.3	95.8	74.5	86.2	96.4	74.1	85.9	96.4
35-44	81.1	91.0	96.6	72.0	81.6	92.2	77.3	86.5	94.1
45-54	81.8	87.0	94.8	72.1	83.0	93.8	76.1	89.3	97.0
55-64	70.8	80.6	97.7	74.7	84.0	96.1	75.5	86.3	97.2
≥65	76.2	85.7	100.0	73.3	76.9	94.1	78.3	86.4	94.2
Educational level									
0-8	79.8	83.9	95.0	75.8	83.9	94.6	74.9	81.7	91.2
9-11	78.8	87.8	95.4	76.8	87.1	96.9	70.8	84.7	94.5
12	80.9	92.1	96.7	70.6	82.8	93.9	74.1	85.4	95.6
13-15	81.6	93.3	98.9	68.9	82.8	94.2	67.1	84.0	95.7
≥16	77.0	88.0	97.0	65.7	78.4	92.1	70.3	81.5	93.9

(1) National Survey on Adult Use of Tobacco, PHS.

(2) National Health Interview Survey Smoking Supplement, PHS.

SOURCE: USDHHS (1983).

in smoking among younger women in their early 20s. This increase can, in turn, be explained partly by the movement into their 20s of women who were teenagers in the 1970s when smoking rates among teenage women were increasing, a trend which has already begun to reverse (USDHHS, 1983). This trend, coupled with the tendency for younger smokers to be less successful in their attempts to quit, suggests that, as this cohort of women in their early 20s matures, overall gender differences in the rates of successful smoking cessation will diminish even further.

Jarvis (1984) has recently suggested another, and very different challenge to the claim that women smokers find it harder to give up smoking. Due to methodological difficulties related to the way in which relevant self-reported behavior data has been collected, gender differences in smoking cessation rates may be exaggerated due to the higher percentage of male smokers who cross over to pipe or cigar use, but who describe themselves as former cigarette smokers. Whether or not the reported gender differences in cigarette smoking prevalence and cessation rates over the past two decades have been exaggerated, a great deal remains unanswered that could have significant implications for the control of smoking among women in the future.

We do not know, for example, whether or not physiological or metabolic differences may be at the root of reported gender differences in factors such as negative affect, nervousness, anxiety, or weight gain following smoking cessation. In addition, we know very little about the factors underlying the apparent gender differences in treatment success rates. It should be noted in this regard that these data have been collected from self-selected treatment populations seeking the help of various intervention modalities. This population is likely to be very different from the 85-90% of all successful quitters who are estimated to quit on their own without the aid of an organized intervention (USDHHS, 1983). Very little is known about gender differences among that group which quits on its own. Since the self-reported success rates for adult women have improved since 1970, and since these rates have been nearly indistinguishable from those of men, the observed improvements are likely to be found among the self-quitters. Further research in this area is obviously needed.

We also know very little that would predict which smokers, male or female, benefit from specific forms of treatment in formal intervention programs. A number of factors contribute to this confusion.

For example, relatively little research has been devoted to the study of the effectiveness of different smoking cessation techniques for different subgroups of smokers. Aversive conditioning might be more effective for those who smoke primarily for positive reinforcement, whereas desensitization or relaxation techniques might be more appropriate for those who smoke primarily to control anxiety. Since most treatment effectiveness studies have not attempted to categorize smokers by either meaningful subgroups or by sex, potentially significant individual variations have been obscured. The fact that many intervention strategies utilize multicomponent treatment approaches serves to compound the problem. Furthermore, even when program success rates are reported, the critical issue of which participants, male or female, actually complied with the intervention protocol is seldom addressed (Leventhal et al., 1984). Many of those quitters who are counted as program "successes" may have not used the intended techniques at all. This issue is highly complex and obviously multidimensional. Until more is known about the idiopathic relationships between specific smokers and specific cessation approaches, conclusions regarding gender differences should be made with caution. Further research in this area could result in an improved understanding of optimal cessation approaches for both women and men.

REFERENCES

American Institute of Public Opinion (Gallup). The Gallup Poll Public Opinion, *1935–1971 Series*, 477–1501: *1972–1977 Series*, 274–1203.

Bozzetti, L. P. Group Psychotherapy with Addicted Smokers. (1972). *Psychotherapy and Psychosomatics, 20*, 172–175.

Burns, B. H. (1969). Chronic Chest Disease, Personality, and Success in Stopping Cigarette Smoking. *British Journal of Preventive and Social Medicine, 23(1)*, 23–27.

Cherry, N., & Kiernan, K. (1976). Personality Scores and Smoking Behavior. *British Journal of Preventive and Social Medicine, 30*, 123–131.

Garrod, J. W., & Jenner, P. (1975). The Metabolism of Tobacco Alkaloids. In: Hayes, W. J., Jr. (Ed.). Essays in Toxicology, New York: Academic Press.

Graham, H. (1976). Smoking in Pregnancy: The attitudes of expectant Mothers. *Social Science and Medicine, 10*, 399–405.

Guilford, J. (1972). Group Treatment Versus Individual Initiative in the Cessation of Smoking. *Journal of Applied Psychology, 56*, 162–167.

Haenszel, W., Shimkin, M. B., & Miller, H. P. (1956). Tobacco Smoking Patterns in the United States. U.S. Department of Health, Education, and Welfare, Public Health Service, *Monograph No. 45*.

Hammond, E. C., & Garfinkel, L. (1968). Changes in Cigarette Smoking 1959–1965, *American Journal of Public Health, 58*(1), 30–45.

Harris, J. E., (1979, January). Cigarette Smoking in the United States, 1950–1978. *Smoking and Health, A Report of the Surgeon General*, U.S. Department of Health, Education, and Welfare, Public Health Service, Office of the Assistant Secretary of Health, Office on Smoking and Health, A1–A29.

Howe, H. (1984, May–June). An Historical Review of Women, Smoking, and Advertising. *Health Education*, 3–9.

Ikard, F. F., & Tomkins, S. (1973). The Experience of Affect as a Determinant of Smoking Behavior. A Series of Validity Studies. *Journal of Abnormal Psychology, 81(2)*, 173–181.

Jackson, E. L. (1950, November). Trends in the consumption of tobacco products, United States, 1900–1950. *Journal of Farm Economics, 32*, (4: Part 2), 881–883.

Jarvis, M. (1984). Gender and Smoking: Do Women Really Find it Harder to Give Up? *British Journal of Addiction, 79(4)*, 383–387.

Leventhal, H., Zimmerman, R., & Gutmann, M. (1984). Compliance: A Self-Regulation Perspective. In: W.D. Gentry (Ed.), *Handbook of Behavioral Medicine*. New York: Guilford Press.

Lichtenstein, E., Antonuccio, D., & Rainwater, G. (1977). Unkicking the Habit: The Resumption of Cigarette Smoking. Western Psychological Association, Washington.

Lichtenstein, E., & Brown, R. A. (1980). Smoking Cessation Methods: Review and Recommendations. In W. R. Miller (Ed.), *The Addictive Behaviors*, New York: Pergamon Press.

Peterson, D. I., Lonergan, L. H., Hardinge, M. G., & Teel, C. W. (1968). Results of a Stop-Smoking Program. *Archives of Environmental Health, 16(2)*, 211–214.

Russell, M. A. H. (1970). Effect of Electric Aversion on Cigarette Smoking. *British Medical Journal, 1(5688)*, 82–86.

Schievelbein, H., & Heinemann, G., Loschenkohl, K., Troll, C., & Schlegel, J. (1978). Metabolic Aspects of Smoking Behavior. In: Thornton, R. E. (Ed.), *Smoking Behavior*, Edinburgh: Churchill Livingstone.

Shiffman, S. M. (1979). The Tobacco Withdrawal Syndrome. In: Krasnegor, N. A. (Ed.). Cigarette Smoking as a Dependence Process. Department of Health, Education, and Welfare, Public Health Service, Alcohol, Drug Abuse, and Mental Health Health Administration, National Institute on Drug Abuse, *Research Monograph 23*, 158–185.

Tennant, R. B. (1950). *The American Cigarette Industry*. New Haven: Yale University Press.

Trahair, R. C. S. (1967). Giving Up Cigarettes: 222 Case Studies. *Medical Journal of Australia, 1*, 929–932.

U.S. Department of Commerce, Bureau of the Census. (1975). Historical Statistics of the United States, Colonial Times to the Present.

U.S. Department of Health, Education, and Welfare. (1964). Smoking and Health, Report of the Advisory Committee to the Surgeon General of the Public Health Service, Public Health Service, *1103*, 387pp.

U.S. Department of Health, Education, and Welfare. (1969). Use of Tobacco Practices, Attitudes, Knowledge, and Beliefs. U. S. Fall 1964 and Spring 1966. Department of Health, Education, and Welfare, National Clearinghouse for Smoking and Health, 807pp.

U.S. Department of Health, Education, and Welfare. (1970). Changes in Cigarette Smoking Habits between 1965–1966. Vital and Health Statistics, Series *10*, No. 59.

U.S. Department of Health, Education, and Welfare. (1973). Adult Use of Tobacco 1970. Department of Health, Education, and Welfare, National Clearinghouse for Smoking and Health, (HSM) *73–8727*.

U.S. Department of Health, Education, and Welfare. (1976). 1975 Study of Cigarette Smoking Among Four Health Professional Groups in the U. S.: Basic Tabulations. Department of Health, Education, and Welfare, Center for Disease Control, Bureau of Health Education, National Clearinghouse for Smoking and Health.

U.S. Department of Health, Education, and Welfare. (1979). Changes in Cigarette Consumption and Current Smoking Practices Among Adults: U. S., 1978. Public Health Service, National Center for Health Statistics, *52*, 1–16.

U.S. Department of Health and Human Services. (1979). The Health Consequences of Smoking for Women: A Report of the Surgeon General. U.S. Department of Health and Human Services, Public Health Service, Office of the Assistant Secretary for Health, Office on Smoking and Health.

U.S. Department of Health and Human Services. (1982). The Health Consequences of Smoking: A Report of the Surgeon General. U.S. Department of Health and Human Services, Public Health Service, Office of the Assistant Secretary for Health, Office on Smoking and Health, 302 pp.

U.S. Department of Health and Human Services. (1983). The Health Consequences of Smoking: Cardiovascular Disease. A Report of the Surgeon General. U.S. Department of Health and Human Services, Public Health Service, Office of the Assistant Secretary for Health, Office on Smoking and Health, 378 pp.

Wilhelmsen, L. (1968). One Year's Experience in an Antismoking Clinic. *Scandinavian Journal of Respiratory Diseases, 49(4)*, 251–259.

Yankelovitch, Skelly, & White, Inc. (1977). A Study of Cigarette Smoking among Teen-age Girls and Young Women. Summary of the Findings. Department of Health, Education, and Welfare, Public Health Service, National Institutes of Health, National Cancer Institute, DHEW (NIH) No. *77–1203*.

Smokeless Tobacco and Cancer in Women: Implications for Cancer Research

Deborah M. Winn, PhD
Linda Williams Pickle, PhD

ABSTRACT. Smokeless tobacco, particularly snuff, is a recognized risk factor for cancer of the oral cavity. This conclusion rests in large part on epidemiologic studies of oral cancer in women, especially in the American South, where the oral cancer death rate in females has been high. The research focus on studies of women led to the identification of the hazards from smokeless tobacco use; the strategies used are broadly applicable to studies of the etiology of other cancers in both women and men. High levels of nitrosamines, which are potent carcinogens, are found in smokeless tobacco products. Steps should be taken to reverse the alarming increase in their use by men and boys. More research attention also should be directed to understanding new emerging trends in oral cancer mortality among women.

INTRODUCTION

Research initiated to elucidate the causes of the longstanding "epidemic" of mouth cancer among Southern U.S. women has uncovered compelling evidence linking smokeless tobacco use to cancer in humans. Smokeless tobacco includes chewing tobacco and snuff, which is placed between the gum and either the lip or cheek. Snuff may be a finely ground powder ("dry" snuff) or finely cut with a higher moisture content ("moist"). Chewing tobacco is coarser in texture and is sold in the form of plugs, loose leaves in a pouch, or, uncommonly, in a braid. In the epidemiologic investigations of the epidemic of mouth cancer among women in the south, some of the

Deborah M. Winn is with the Survey and Planning and Development Branch, Divison of Health Examination Statistics, National Center for Health Statistics, Hyattsville, MD 20872.
Linda Williams Pickle is with the Division of Cancer Etiology, Environmental Epidemiology Branch, National Cancer Institute, Bethesda, MD 20892.

special characteristics often common to populations of women (e.g., until recently, a lower prevalence of cigarette smoking) were critical in pointing to and confirming analytically that the agent responsible for the high oral cancer death rates in the South was smokeless tobacco. This paper will describe trends and research on smokeless tobacco and mouth cancer and will show that the investigation of the link between smokeless tobacco and mouth cancer is but one example of many studies among women which have yielded important knowledge about cancer etiology in both men and women.

HISTORY AND PAST TRENDS IN USE OF SMOKELESS TOBACCO

Both smokeless and smoking tobacco were introduced by Indians in Central and South America to European explorers in the sixteenth century, who in turn introduced tobacco to other cultures throughout the world. Although both men and women have used smokeless tobacco for centuries, a few women throughout history have received considerable notoriety for their enthusiasm about snuff inhaling. Among them are Catherine de Medici who hoped its putative medicinal properties would help her sick son, and Queen Charlotte, wife of England's King George III, a devoted snuff inhaler who was sometimes referred to as "Snuffy Charlotte."[1] Snuff inhaling by English colonists in America was not uncommon, but most Americans who adopted the habit favored taking smokeless tobacco by mouth rather than inhaling it.[2] A major peak in use in the U.S. occurred from 1830 to the early 20th century. Thereafter, the use of smokeless tobacco declined markedly until the 1970s[1] in all but a few areas and groups in the U.S. One segment of the U.S. population in which snuff use continued to be an important custom was Southern women.[2] Since the 1970s the popularity of chewing tobacco and snuff has increased markedly,[3] although much of the increase in use is apparent in males, and not females.

SMOKELESS TOBACCO AS A CAUSE OF CANCER

The link between the use of smokeless tobacco and cancer also has a long history, beginning in 1761 when a report of nasal tumors in heavy users of snuff was reported.[4] Knowledge of the association between oral use of unsmoked tobacco and cancer dates to 1837 when a tobacco chewer with tongue cancer was described.[5] Reports throughout the 20th century have described oral cancers among smokeless tobacco users which had arisen precisely where the tobacco quid was placed routinely.[6] Many of these reports came from clinicians in the Southern U.S.; several investigators remarked that, unlike populations elsewhere, the patients with mouth cancer were more likely to be women than men.[7] This inversion of the sex ratio typically seen for this cancer, roughly 4 men to every woman who died of oral cancer,[8] suggested to these investigators that an important etiologic factor was involved.

Field studies conducted in these high risk areas also have linked smokeless tobacco use to oral cancer. We conducted an epidemiologic study of oral cancer among women in North Carolina[9] to investigate reasons for the unusually high oral cancer death rate among Southern white women. Included as cases in the study were 232 women who had been hospitalized with oral or pharyngeal cancer at 5 North Carolina hospitals between 1975–78 or who had died from oral and pharynx cancer in 67 counties of that state. Each case was matched to two controls by age, race and area of residence. The women themselves (or the next-of-kin of deceased subjects) were interviewed in their homes using a structured questionnaire eliciting information about a variety of factors including tobacco habits.

Among the non-cigarette smokers, snuff use was 4 times more common in the cases than controls. Among the non-smoking women with cancer of the buccal mucosa and gum, where the smokeless tobacco is placed routinely, the relative risks were even higher: from 13-fold for less than 50 years of use to almost 50 fold for very long term use (i.e., 50 years or more). Black women and white women who also smoked cigarettes had lower relative risks because of their lower intensity and duration of snuff use. Smoking was also an important risk factor in this study with an effect independent of that for snuff. We concluded that the unusual mortality pattern among women in the area could be accounted for by the longstanding custom of using smokeless tobacco.

Other studies conducted in the U.S., especially in the South, and in Scandinavia where the oral use of smokeless tobacco is also common show that oral cancer patients are several times more likely to use smokeless tobacco than controls.[6] One other study in addition to our own found that the relative risk increased with greater use of smokeless tobacco (measured, like ''packyears'', by frequency of use times duration of use).[10] The epidemiologic findings are supported by laboratory research which shows that nitrosamines are extractable from smokeless tobacco in amounts higher than those found in any other consumer product, including tobacco smoke. These tobacco-specific nitrosamines have been shown to produce cancers, typically in the esophagus and lung, in laboratory animals.[11] Elsewhere in the world, the use of smokeless tobacco is very popular, especially tobacco mixed with other ingredients (e.g., areca "betel" nut). These tobacco mixtures are associated with enormous increases in oral cancer risk[12] and account in part for the extremely high incidence and death rates for these cancers in India[13] and the Pacific Islands. Smokeless tobacco use is associated with the presence of leukoplakia, or white patches in the mouth.[14] Certain types of leukoplakia are associated with an increased oral cancer risk[15] and leukoplakia is frequently present in oral cancer patients with a longterm smokeless tobacco habit.[5] The evidence that smokeless tobacco causes oral cancer is summarized in Table 1.

THE UNIQUE CONTRIBUTION TO CANCER ETIOLOGY FROM EPIDEMIOLOGIC RESEARCH OF WOMEN

Special studies of women and cancer sometimes have been particularly successful in advancing our understanding of cancer

TABLE 1

EVIDENCE SMOKELESS TOBACCO CAUSES MOUTH CANCER

Many reports have described patients whose mouth cancer arose precisely where tobacco had been placed routinely.

The association is almost always evident in case-control and cohort studies in various parts of the U.S. and Scandinavia.

Other risk factors for mouth cancer besides smokeless tobacco (e.g., smoking) can be ruled out in some studies.

Two studies show that the relative risks increase with heavier use of smokeless tobacco.

Nitrosamines, which cause cancer in laboratory animals, are found in very high levels in smokeless tobacco.

Smokeless tobacco, usually taken with other ingredients, also is related to oral cancer risk in Asian populations.

Smokeless tobacco is associated with leukoplakia (i.e., white patches in the mouth) which is also associated with an increase risk of mouth cancer.

etiology in men and women and have broad implications for health research in general. The study of cancer risks associated with smokeless tobacco and our case-control study of oral cancer in North Carolina[9] demonstrate some of the special contributions which may be derived from studies of cancer in women. One benefit is the wealth of information obtained by contrasting, by means of the sex ratio, the mortality or morbidity experience of men and women. The sex ratio is the ratio of the incidence or mortality rate in men versus women. The unusual predominance of oral cancer in Southern women[7] was one clue leading to more definitive research on smokeless tobacco and cancer. Other aberrations in the typical sex ratio for oral cancer have been observed, which also pointed to the action of a habit with a major effect on oral cancer risk. In one area in the Indian state of Andhra Pradesh, women with oral cancer in the roof of the mouth outnumber men by 3 to 2.[16] The unusual habit of reverse smoking, in which a homemade cigarette is smoked with the lit end in the mouth, is practiced most frequently by women in the area and accounts for the excess oral cancer among them.

For other cancers, the sex ratio also has been an important clue to etiology. Previously the high ratio of rates of lung cancer in men versus women was cited to show that women were intrinsically less susceptible to lung cancer compared to men.[17] However, the ratio of lung cancer mortality rates in men versus women was 3.6 to 1 in 1976–80, a drop from the previous ratios of 5–7 to 1 in the 5 year interval from 1950–54 to 1970–1975,[18] implying an environmental, not genetic, influence. This fact, coupled with the observation that, given the same smoking patterns, the magnitude of the relative risk associated with cigarette smoking is similar for men and women,[19] suggests that both sexes are equally susceptible to lung cancer due to smoking.

Valuable information may often be obtained from studying groups at lower baseline risks and, for some cancers, populations of women constitute such a group. Smoking is a well-established and potent risk factor for oral cancer.[20] Yet in the North Carolina study, 57% of the women were not cigarette smokers, a proportion higher than that in large studies of men with these cancers.[21] Because smoking was not universal in the case series, it was possible to examine other potential etiologic factors, especially smokeless tobacco use, as well as other factors (e.g., diet[22]) while eliminating the potential confounding role of smoking. In contrast eliminating smoking as a confounder in the evaluation of the relationship between chewing tobacco (a "male" habit) and oral cancer has proven more difficult since epidemiologic studies tend to find that male chewers also smoke.

This same principle, identifying study groups at low risk, also applies in research on other cancers. Lung cancer risk associated with passive smoking is one important issue that has been addressed successfully by studies of women otherwise at low risk of lung cancer. In Japan Hirayama has shown that non-smoking women whose husbands smoked were twice as likely to die of lung cancer than non-smokers with husbands who did not smoke.[23] It was possible to make this finding because Japanese women have relatively low baseline levels of lung cancer: the proportion of women who smoke is low and employment at jobs associated with exposure to lung carcinogens is rare. These characteristics make detection of the effects of passive smoking possible because other contributors to lung cancer risk are at low levels.

The sequence of research leading to the North Carolina study is an example of the progression of epidemiologic research. The National Cancer Institute (NCI) studies began with maps of cancer mortality by county or state economic area.[8] Inspection of the maps revealed the area of high cancer mortality from mouth and throat cancer among white women in the Southeastern United States (Figure 1). The magnitude of the oral cancer death rates as well as the discrepancy in rates for men and women led the NCI researchers to examine the geographic patterns in more detail,[24] leading to estimates about the magnitude of the excess mortality and observations concerning county demographic and industrial correlates of mortality. White women in the Southeast were estimated to have death rates from oral cancer about 90% above U.S. rates in rural areas and 30% in urban areas. These hypothesis-generating activities led to the analytic study of the North Carolina population described above.[9] This sequence of hypothesis-generating to hypothesis-testing studies, while not unique to studies of women, is typical of epidemiologic research and is applicable in other areas of health research.

CURRENT TRENDS IN ORAL CANCER DEATH RATES

Recently cancer mortality maps for the thirty year period 1950–80 have been prepared[18] which show trends in cancer death rates over calendar time. The trends for oral cancer by sex (Figure 2) show

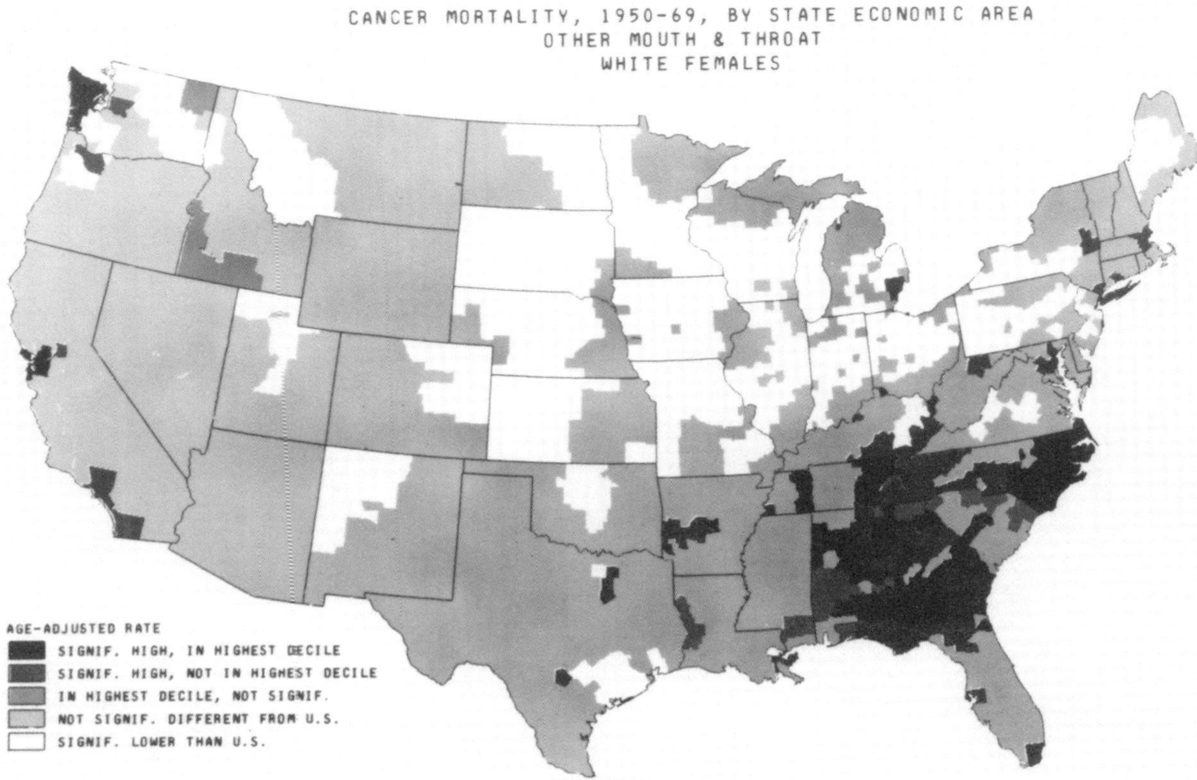
CANCER MORTALITY, 1950-69, BY STATE ECONOMIC AREA
OTHER MOUTH & THROAT
WHITE FEMALES
AGE-ADJUSTED RATE
SIGNIF. HIGH, IN HIGHEST DECILE
SIGNIF. HIGH, NOT IN HIGHEST DECILE
IN HIGHEST DECILE, NOT SIGNIF.
NOT SIGNIF. DIFFERENT FROM U.S.
SIGNIF. LOWER THAN U.S.

FIGURE 1

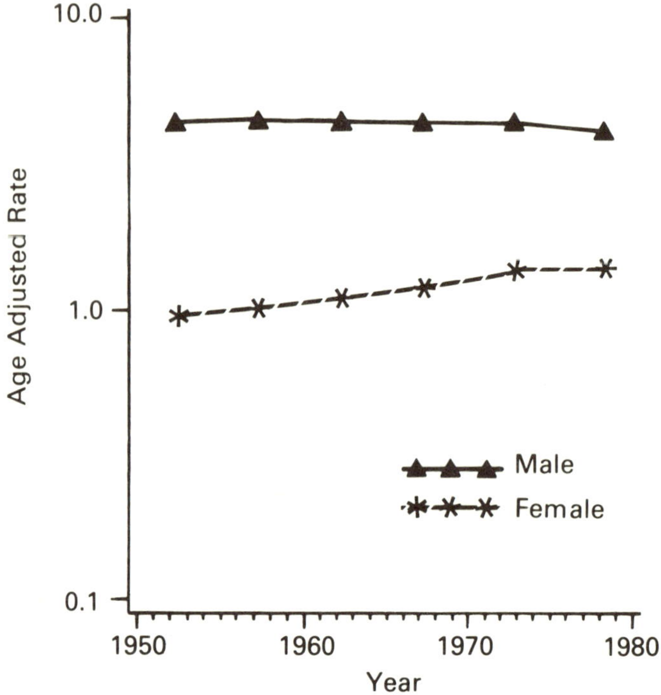

FIGURE 2. Age-Adjusted (1960 U.S. Standard) Mortality Rates for Cancer of the Oral Cavity by Gender and Time Period

that the age-adjusted death rates for women increased by an average of 8.4% in each time period, rising from 0.98 per 100,000 in 1950–54 to 1.43 per 100,000 in 1976–80. Men experienced a slight decline over time dropping by 0.8% on average in each 5-year period. This rate of increase in women is in the top third of increases in the major cancer sites, but the most striking feature is the discrepancy by sex with rates for women rising and those for men dropping slightly. While the death rates for men exceeded those for women in every time period, the ratio of death rates in men versus women is declining as the rates among women increase.

When the mortality rates for women are ascertained by geographic area and time period, more interesting changes are observed. As shown in the map for 1970–1980 (Figure 3), areas which have recently emerged as having the highest oral cancer death rates include portions of California and Florida.[18] Oral and pharynx cancer death rates for women by decade from 1950–59 to 1970–79 remained stable in North Carolina (1.8, 1.7, 1.8 per 100,000 per year for 1950–59, 1960–6, and 1970–79, respectively), while U.S. rates increased (1.1, 1.2, 1.5). In contrast, oral and pharynx cancer rates in California women nearly doubled (1.1, 1.5, 2.1) and, by the 1970–79 decade, exceeded North Carolina and U.S. rates. Other areas with marked increases over time in female oral cancer death rates include the District of Columbia (1.1, 2.1, 3.3), Florida (1.1, 1.6, 1.9), Maryland(1.1, 1.3, 2.0), Nevada (1.0, 1.6, 2.1) and New Hampshire (0.9, 1.2, 1.7).[25]

CURRENT TRENDS IN SMOKELESS TOBACCO USE IN GIRLS AND WOMEN

In the North Carolina study population women of all ages used smokeless tobacco; however, use of the product was less common in the younger study subjects.[26] In addition, sales of dry snuff, the form most popular among the North Carolina study subjects, have declined over time.[27] Currently, 2% of girls 12–17 years old in the U.S. have tried smokeless tobacco at least once in the past year according to preliminary data from a recently completed survey conducted by the National Institute for Drug Abuse.[28] Estimates from local surveys also suggest that the prevalence of girls who ever tried smokeless tobacco or who define themselves as ''users'' was less than 3%[29,30,31] with one exception.[32] One survey[33] found no girls using the product. When they do try the product, girls seem less likely to sustain the habit; one study of 7th, 9th and 10th graders found that 20% of girls surveyed had tried smokeless tobacco, but on average only a very small percentage (0.7–2.4% depending on grade) used it daily.[32]

In contrast, smokeless tobacco use is popular in boys and young men. The national rates suggest that 16% of boys 12–17 years old have used smokeless tobacco in the past year,[28] and one third of this 16% used it at least once per week. Surveys in state and local populations find wide variation. At the extreme one study reported that two-thirds to three-quarters of boys in the 7th, 9th, and 10th grades had tried smokeless tobacco at least once;[32] in the same study

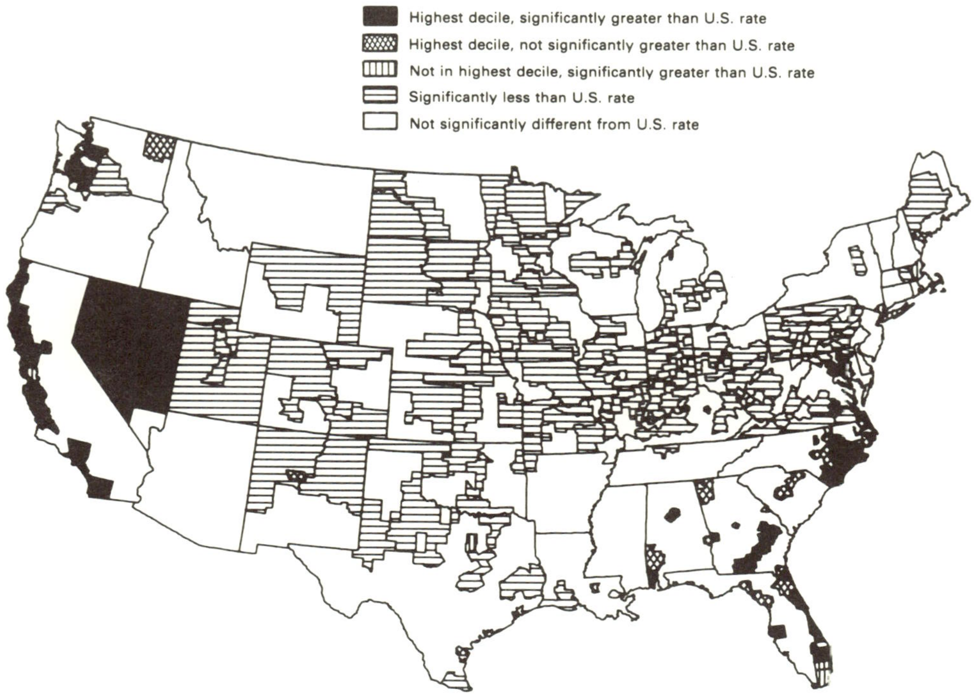

Figure 3. Cancer Mortality Rates, 1970-80, by State Economic Area
Oral Cavity, White Females
U.S. Rate = 1.4/100,000

9–23% (depending on grade) were using the product daily. Use often starts at a very young age in both boys and girls; one study of kindergarten pupils in Arkansas reported that 21.4% had tried smokeless tobacco and another reported that 66% of the smokeless users started at age 12 or younger.[34]

FUTURE RESEARCH AND PUBLIC HEALTH INTERVENTIONS

Other health effects associated with smokeless tobacco include gingival (i.e., gum) recession and tobacco dependence.[28] For pregnant women the risks might include low birth weight and length and other abnormalities, since these outcomes have been noted in Asian Indian women with a tobacco chewing habit;[35] however, the applicability of these findings is unclear because the quids probably contained other toxic constituents in addition to the tobacco. Because young women and girls currently seem to have low rates of use of smokeless tobacco, the future contribution of smokeless tobacco to cancer and other health consequences among women fortunately may be small. Efforts should be made to keep the prevalence of use of smokeless tobacco in girls low. Advertising for smokeless tobacco typically is directed to boys and men, rather than girls[36] and may account in part for the difference in use by sex. As was pointed out at the recent NIH Consensus Conference (January 13–15, 1986), girls may also play an important role in discouraging use among male friends by emphasizing the aesthetically distasteful aspects of smokeless tobacco by boys (e.g., expectoration, appearance of teeth).

Death rates from oral and pharynx cancer in North Carolina have remained fairly constant over time, but substantial increases in rates elsewhere (e.g., California and Florida) have begun to surpass the persistently high rates in the Southeast. It is probable that these trends are related more to smoking and drinking habits than to smokeless tobacco, however. Smokeless tobacco is most strongly associated with cancer of the buccal mucosa (cheek) and gum,[9] whereas smoking seems to have a greater impact on the risk of pharynx cancer than it has on mouth cancer.[20] Interestingly mortality data (Pickle, unpublished) suggests that buccal mucosal and gum cancer accounted for 46% of all deaths from mouth/pharynx cancer in North Carolina from 1969–73, but only 22% of mouth/pharynx cancers in California. Conversely, only 7% of the mouth/pharynx cancers in North

Carolina occurred in the pharynx, in sharp contrast to 23% in California. One could speculate that these differentials are due to the use of smokeless tobacco in North Carolina and smoking on the West Coast; increasing mortality due to smoking might be reflected in an increasing rate of death over time due to pharynx cancer (and possibly other mouth cancer sites exclusive of the gum and buccal mucosa). Thus, it will be important to monitor trends in oral and pharynx cancer death rates, especially by subtypes, and to investigate further reasons for the increases in oral cancer mortality among women.

Steps should be taken to stem the use of smokeless tobacco in boys, since the rates of mouth cancer may rise in the future as a consequence of the increasing use of smokeless tobacco. In addition as boys become habituated to smokeless tobacco, they might switch to smoking as they grow older.

Lessons learned in epidemiologic research on smokeless tobacco, especially from studies of women, have proven critically important in evaluating the role of oral cancer risk factors and in explaining the geographical pattern of oral cancer occurrence. Our knowledge of the health consequences of these habits should inspire serious efforts to counteract the current epidemic of smokeless tobacco use in men and boys. Further research on cancer conducted in populations of women is likely to provide a wealth of information about cancer and its etiology in both sexes.

NOTES

1. Christen, A.G., Swanson, B.Z., Glover, E.D., & Henderson, A.H. (1982). Smokeless tobacco: The folklore and social history of snuffing, sneezing, dipping, and chewing. *J.A.D.A.* 105: 821–829.

2. The Tobacco Institute, Inc. (1959). The snuff industry; the chewing tobacco industry. Washington, DC: The Tobacco Institute.

3. Shelton, A. (1982, August). Smokeless sales continue to climb. *Tobacco Reporter*, pp. 59–60.

4. Redmond, D.E. (1970). Tobacco and cancer: The first clinical report, 1761. *N. Engl. J. Med.* 282: 18–23.

5. Wynder, E.L. (1976) A corner of history: John Collins Warren, 1778–1856. *Prev. Med.* 5: 317–319.

6. International Agency for Research on Cancer. (1985). IARC Monographs on the Evaluation of the Carcinogenic Risk of Chemicals to Humans—Tobacco Habits Other Than Smoking; Betel Quid; and Some Related Nitrosamines, vol. 37. Lyon: International Agency for Research on Cancer.

7. Brown, R.L., Suh, J.M., Scarborough, J.E., Wilkins, S.A., & Smith, R.R. (1965). Snuff-dippers' intraoral cancer: Clinical characteristics and response to therapy. *Cancer* 18: 2–13.

8. Mason, T.J., McKay, F.W., Hoover, R., Blot, W.J., & Fraumeni, J.F. Jr. (1975). Atlas of cancer mortality for U.S. counties, 1950–69. Washington, DC: Government Printing Office. (NIH 75–780).

9. Winn, D.M., Blot, W.J., Shy, C.M., Pickle, L.W., Toledo, A., & Fraumeni, J.F., Jr. (1981). Snuff dipping and oral cancer among women in the Southern United States. *New Engl. J. Med.* 304: 745–749.

10. Williams, R.R., & Horm, J.W. (1977). Association of cancer sites with tobacco and alcohol consumption and socioeconomic status of patients; Interview study from the Third National Cancer Survey. *J. Natl Cancer Inst.* 58: 525–547.

11. Hoffmann, D., & Hecht, S.S. (1985). Nicotine-derived N-nitrosamines and tobacco-related cancer: Current status and future directions. *Cancer Res.* 45: 935–944.

12. Gupta, P.C., Pindborg, J.J., & Mehta, F.S. (1982). Comparison of carcinogenicity of betel quid with and without tobacco: An epidemiologic review. *Ecol. Dis.* 1: 213–219.

13. Waterhouse, J., Muir, C., Correa, P., et al., (eds.). (1976). Cancer Incidence in 5 Continents, Vol. III. WHO Publication #15. Lyon, International Agency for Research on Cancer.

14. Peacock, E.E., Greenberg, B.G., & Brawley, B.W. (1960). The effect of snuff and tobacco on the production of oral carcinoma: An experimental and epidemiologic study. *Ann. Surg.* 151: 542–550.

15. Silverman, S., Gorsky, M., & Lozada, F. (1984). Oral leukoplakia and malignant transformation. *Cancer* 53: 563–568.

16. Reddy, C.R.R.M., Prahlad, D., & Ramulu, C. (1975). Incidence of oral cancer with particular reference to hard palate cancer in 1 million population in the district of Visakhapatnam. *Indian J. Cancer* 12: 72–76.

17. Ashley, D.J.B., & Davies, H.D. (1969). Lung cancer in women. *Thorax* 24:446–450.

18. Pickle, L.W., Mason, T.J., Howard, N., Hoover, R., & Fraumeni, J.F., Jr. (in press). Atlas of U.S. Cancer Mortality Among Whites, 1950–1980. Washington, DC: U.S. Government Printing Office.

19. Lubin, J.H., & Blot, W.J. (1984). Assessment of lung cancer risk factors by histologic type. *J. Natl. Cancer Inst.* 73: 383–389.

20. Office on Smoking and Health, PHS. (1982). Health consequences of smoking—Cancer. Washington, DC: U.S. Government Printing Office.

21. Keller, A.Z., & Terris, M. (1965). The association of alcohol and tobacco with cancers of the mouth and pharynx. *Amer. J. Public Health* 55: 1578–1585.

22. Winn, D.M., Ziegler, R.G., Pickle, L.W., Gridley, G., Blot, W.J., & Hoover, R.N. (1984). Diet in the etiology of oral and pharynx cancer among women from the Southern U.S. *Cancer Res* 44: 1216–1222.

23. Hirayama, T. (1981). Non-smoking wives of heavy smokers have a higher risk of lung cancer: A study in Japan. *Br. Med. J.* 282: 183–185; 283: 1466.

24. Blot, W.J., & Fraumeni, J.F. Jr. (1977). Geographic patterns of oral cancer in the U.S.: etiologic implications. *J. Chr. Dis.* 30: 745–757.

25. Riggan, W.B., Van Bruggen, J., Acquavella, J.F., Beaubier, J., & Mason, T.J. (1983). U.S. Cancer Mortality Rates and Trends, 1950–1979. Washington, DC, U.S. Government Printing Office, (EPA–600/1–83–015a).

26. Winn, D.M. (1980). Oral and pharyngeal cancer in relation to tobacco use, alcohol, and occupation. Ph.D. Dissertation, 1980. University of North Carolina, Chapel Hill, NC.

27. Maxwell, J.C. (1982, July 23). *Tobacco International*, Table p. 125.

28. National Institutes of Health Consensus Conference. (1986). Health implications of smokeless tobacco use. *JAMA* 255: 1045–1048.

29. Poulson, T.C., Lindenmuth, J.E., & Greer, R.O. Jr. (1984). A comparison of the use of smokeless tobacco in rural and urban teenagers. *CA: A Cancer Journal for Clinicians 34*: 248–261.

30. Marty, P.J., McDermott, R.J., & Williams, T. (1986). Patterns of smokeless tobacco use in a population of high school students. *AJPH* 76: 190–192.

31. Hunter, S.M., Croft, J.B., Burke, G.L., Parker, F.C., Webber, L.S., & Berenson, G.S. (1986). Longitudinal patterns of cigarette smoking and smokeless tobacco use in youth: The Bogalusa Heart Study. *Am J. Public Health* 76: 193–195.

32. Lichtenstein, E., Severson, H.H., Friedman, L.S., & Ary, D.V. (in press). Chewing tobacco use by adolescents: Prevalence and relation to cigarette smoking. Addictive Behaviors.

33. Guggenheimer, J., Zullo, T.G., Kruper, D.C., & Verbin, R.S. (1986). Changing trends of tobacco use in a teenage population in Western Pennsylvania. *Am J. Public Health* 76: 196–197.

34. Young, M., & Williamson, D. (1985). Correlates of use of expected use of smokeless tobacco among kindergarten children. *Psych. Rep.* 56: 63–66.

35. Verm, R.C., Chansoriya, M., & Kaul, K.K. (1983). Effect of tobacco chewing by mothers on fetal outcome. *Indian Ped.* 20: 105–111.

36. Wallis, C. (1985, July 15). Into the mouths of babes. *Time Magazine*, P. 68.

Health Risks of Passive Smoking

Cheri M. Papier, MPH, MS
Steven D. Stellman, PhD

ABSTRACT. Passive or involuntary smoking is the inhalation of smoke which escapes directly into the air from the lit end of a burning cigarette. This unfiltered smoke contains the same toxic components of the mainstream smoke inhaled directly by the smoker, including numerous carcinogens, many in greater concentrations. It has long been known that exposure to this type of smoke leads to increased respiratory and other adverse health conditions in non-smokers, especially children. During the past five years, evidence has been accumulating that risk of lung cancer is also higher, particularly in non-smoking women whose husbands smoke. Despite uncertainties and differences in interpretation of various cancer studies, there is ample justification for public health measures now in place or proposed, such as restriction or elimination of smoking in the workplace and in public places.

INTRODUCTION

Use of tobacco ranks as one of the most serious health problems among American women. Elsewhere in this issue Virginia Ernster has pointed out that cigarette smoking accounts for over 50,000 deaths per year from cancer of the lung, larynx, esophagus, bladder, and other sites (Ernster, 1986), and Deborah Winn and Linda Pickle recount the evidence linking cancer of the mouth with use of smokeless tobacco, such as snuff (Winn and Pickle, 1986).

Both the Ernster and Winn-Pickle papers deal with the lethal effects of tobacco on the woman who uses it. It is increasingly recognized that tobacco use can harm others besides those who consume it directly. This paper summarizes the effects on individuals of exposure to the cigarette smoke of others, with particular attention

Cheri M. Papier is with the Department of Preventive and Social Medicine, Sackler School of Medicine, Tel Aviv University, Tel Aviv 69978 Israel. Steven D. Stellman is Assistant Vice President for Epidemiology, American Cancer Society, 4 West 35th Street, New York, NY 10001.

to possible increase in cancer risk to adult women exposed to the cigarette smoke of others, but who are not themselves smokers.

Non-cancer effects are also briefly mentioned, especially on children and the unborn, in order to emphasize the secondary impact on women, who are primarily responsible for protecting the health of their offspring and caring for them when sick (see also papers by Feldman and Hach in this issue); they are also mentioned to demonstrate that passive smoking carries with it well-established health risks for outcomes other than cancer. These other outcomes have been under investigation for several decades, whereas the earliest cancer study was published only five years ago (Hirayama, 1981). Thus, formal investigation of passive smoking and cancer is not as mature a field as other areas of epidemiological investigation.

While methodological uncertainties do not yet permit the absolutely firm conclusion that passive smoking causes cancer in those exposed, evidence in that direction continues to accumulate. The quality of this evidence, even in its currently incomplete state, leaves no doubt about the propriety of public health measures intended to reduce the risks to non-smokers. These administrative measures will also be discussed below.

WHAT IS PASSIVE SMOKING?

Passive smoking, sometimes called involuntary or second-hand smoking, is the inhalation of smoke given off by a burning cigarette, and can result merely from being in the presence of a smoker. Its harmfulness is related to the distinction between mainstream and sidestream smoke. The smoker, of course, is always exposed to mainstream smoke; this emanates from the burning tip of the cigarette and passes through the as-yet unburned tobacco and the cigarette's filtration system before being absorbed in the smoker's respiratory system.

Non-smokers and smokers alike, on the other hand, are both exposed to the sidestream smoke. This is the unfiltered smoke which rises from the lit end of the burning cigarette, whether held in the smoker's mouth or resting untouched in an ashtray. It also includes the smoke exhaled by the smoker.

Sidestream smoke contains most of the toxic components of mainstream smoke, but at significantly higher concentrations. The ratios of sidestream to mainstream concentrations of some of these components have been reported as: ammonia, 73; methylnaphthalene, 28; aniline, 30; benzo(a)pyrene, 3 (USDHEW, 1979); carbon monoxide, 6.8; nicotine, 6.6; tar, 3.5 (Rickert et al., 1984). These ratios are typical of those for many other toxic compounds found in tobacco smoke, such as pyridine, carbon dioxide, acetone, and oxides of nitrogen. Sidestream smoke is also rich in known carcinogens, such as benzene, benz(a)anthracene, and a variety of nicotine-derived nitrosamines (Brunnemann and Hoffmann, 1978). Formaldehyde and acrolein, two components of tobacco smoke which cause eye and nasal irritation, have been found in sidestream smoke at concentrations up to three orders of magnitude above the limit for occupational exposure (Ayer and Yaeger, 1982).

Precise estimation of the degree of individual exposure to sidestream smoke is extremely difficult to make. Exposure to passive smoking depends on the number and type of cigarettes smoked, the room size, degree of ventilation, and smoke residence time. Carefully controlled studies with non-smoking volunteers exposed to sidestream smoke however, have firmly established measurable elevation of both nicotine and cotinine (its major metabolite) in saliva and urine and of cotinine in plasma (Hoffmann et al., 1984). Cotinine concentrations measured in the saliva of school children were strongly correlated with their parents' smoking habits (Jarvis et al.,1985). Such biological monitoring is both difficult and expensive, and cannot provide estimates of exposures in the past. Therefore, much cruder indexes of exposure in the home or work environment must be used in epidemiological studies.

The extent of exposure in specific populations is difficult to measure, and only limited estimates are available. Friedman and colleagues tabulated questionnaire responses of over 37,000 nonsmokers and former smokers who received multiphasic health checkups in 1979 and 1980 through the Kaiser-Permanente Medical Care Program (Friedman et al., 1983). They reported exposure for at least one hour per week in 63.3% of subjects, at least ten hours per week in 34.5%, and exposure of more than 40 hours per week in 15.9% of their subjects.

Even without direct measurements, it can be assumed that significant exposures occur in people's homes, especially to children. Bonham and Wilson (1981) found that 62% of U.S. homes with children in 1970 contained one or more smokers, and 25% contained two or more. It must therefore be assumed that large numbers of children are exposed to passive smoke in their own homes.

HEALTH RISKS FROM PASSIVE SMOKING

Studies of health effects of passive smoking have appeared with increasing frequency since the early 1960s, and now comprise a substantial literature. Even before cancer was suspected as a possible consequence of passive smoking, effects on reproduction and child growth had already been established. For example, babies of smoking mothers weigh an average of 200 g less than those of non-smoking mothers (USDHEW, 1979, p. 8–11; Butler et al., 1972). Higher rates of fetal loss (spontaneous abortion and stillbirth) have been observed in smoking mothers compared to non-smoking mothers (Goujard et al., 1975; Himmelberger et al., 1978; Stein and Kline, 1973). Higher rates of neonatal and perinatal deaths, as well as sudden infant death syndrome, have been reported (Comstock et al., 1971; Kullander and Kallen, 1971). Effects of smoking on the unborn have been reviewed in Surgeon-General's reports (USDHEW, 1979; USDHHS, 1980) and by McIntosh (1984).

Nursing babies are exposed to their mother's cigarette smoke via breast milk as well as in the air (Trundle and Skellern, 1983). Infants exposed to tobacco smoke absorb enough of its constituents to make measurement of urinary cotinine a reliable measure of such exposure (Greenberg et al., 1984). Children of smoking parents have higher rates of pneumonia, bronchitis, and other respiratory symptoms (Lebowitz and Burrows, 1976; Ware et al., 1984; Schenker et al., 1983; Charlton, 1984). They experience higher hospital admission rates for these conditions than do children of non-smoking parents (Harlap and Davies, 1974).

Non-smoking adults also experience conditions resulting from passive inhalation. Reported effects include eye, nose, and throat irritation (Weber, 1984), headaches, dizziness, and nausea (Shephard et al., 1979), aggravation of allergies and asthma (Knight and Breslin, 1985), and impairment of lung function (Kauffmann et al., 1983).

PASSIVE SMOKING AND CANCER IN ADULT WOMEN

An association between lung cancer in women and exposure to their husbands' cigarette smoke was first reported by Hirayama (1981). In a prospective study, Hirayama found approximately a two-fold increase in risk for Japanese women whose husbands smoked a pack or more per day. A case-control study done in Greece appeared at about the same time in which a relative risk of 3.4 was found for wives of men who smoked over 20 cigarettes per day (Trichopoulos et al., 1981, 1983), and an American case-control study reported similar findings (Correa et al., 1983). In all three of these studies there was evidence of a dose-response relationship, based upon varying definitions of dosage.

Since the appearance of those three studies, a number of other investigations have been undertaken. Not all of these later studies confirmed the smoking-lung cancer link with the same degree of consistency as the first three. In the American Cancer Society's 25-state prospective study the rate of lung cancer in women married to husbands who smoked was 1.2 times that of women married to non-smokers; this increase was not statistically significant (Garfinkel, 1981). Kabat and Wynder (1984) reported an association for men but not women exposed to passive smoke at work, and no effect in either wives or husbands exposed to their spouses' smoke. Other studies have reported significant (Garfinkel et al., 1985; Sandler et al., 1985a,b), borderline (Koo et al., 1983) and non-significant results (Chan, 1982; Wu et al., 1985), respectively. In one of the strongest positive studies, Garfinkel et al. (1985) identified 134 cases of lung cancer and 402 controls with colo-rectal cancer from hospital records in New Jersey and Ohio. All were non-smoking women. The relative risk for lung cancer was 2.11 for women whose husbands smoked 20 or more cigarettes per day at home, compared to wives of non-smoking husbands.

Because of the obvious social and economic implications that would result from acceptance of the causal nature of these associations by the scientific-medical community, all passive smoking studies have been subjected to unusually intense scrutiny, and have been heavily criticized for possible methodological shortcomings. In the most extreme case, the president and director of statistics from The Tobacco Institute (U.S.A.) interpreted a trivial arithmetic discrepancy as a "grave" error which raised "serious questions about the study." Other, more credible questions have been raised, and a lively discussion has appeared in the medical literature (Kornegay et al., 1981; Tsokos et al., 1981; Repace, 1984).

The controversy centers mainly about the extreme difficulty of defining exposure or dosage in a meaningful way. For instance, Garfinkel and colleagues found no association when the dosage variable was hours per day of exposure, either during the past 5 or the past 25 years. An equally important finding was that 40% of women with lung cancer initially identified through hospital records as non-smokers or with smoking status unknown turned out to be smokers at some time during their lives, according to interviews. Another 13% did not have primary lung cancer (Garfinkel et al., 1985). Such misclassification is a major potential source of difficulty in passive smoking studies, and could easily dilute or completely obscure a real effect. These and related problems may be responsible for the lack of consistency in studies published to date.

PUBLIC HEALTH MEASURES FOR REDUCING RISKS FROM PASSIVE SMOKING

In the United States today a major effort is under way to reduce the opportunities for passive exposure to cigarette smoke. This effort began as a movement by non-smokers for the right to breathe clean air and was based originally on reports of eye, nose, and throat irritations, headaches, nausea, dizziness, respiratory congestion and other so-called "minor irritations." It has achieved widespread support and gained considerable momentum, so that today the activities of many organizations involve this issue.

The most widespread activity is the establishment of so-called Clean Indoor Air legislation on state and local levels. As of January, 1986, at least eleven states, ten counties, and more than 30 municipalities had some form of legislation in effect. For instance, smoking in both private and governmental workplaces is restricted in Connecticut, Florida, Maine, Minnesota, Montana, Nebraska, New Jersey, and Utah. Restrictions on smoking in governmental workplaces were enacted in Alaska, California, and Hawaii. Local codes govern workers in San Francisco, and Nassau and Suffolk Counties, New York.

The success of clean air legislation is due to the combined efforts of numerous private and public organizations. A major stimulus to this legislative activity is provided by the National Coalition on Smoking Or Health, which includes the American Cancer Society, American Heart Association, and American Lung Association. Smaller organizations also play key roles, including the California Non-Smokers' Rights Foundation, ASH (Action on Smoking and Health), and GASP (Group Action against Smoking Pollution). Because of the activities of these and other groups, clean air legislation either exists or has been introduced in nearly every state. In addition, a growing number of private businesses now restrict areas where employees may smoke. These firms include Pacific Northwest Bell, Stride Rite Corp., and Boeing Corp.

A second strategy to assert non-smokers' rights to breathe clean air involves direct lawsuits against employers. In 1976, Donna Shimp, an employee of New Jersey Bell Telephone Company, obtained a court injunction ordering Bell to provide a workplace free of cigarette smoke for its non-smoking employees (Shimp v. New Jersey Bell Telephone Company, New Jersey Superior Court, Chancery Division, Para. 21, 421, December 20, 1976). The Court stated in its ruling

> . . . The company already has in effect a rule that cigarettes are not to be smoked around telephone equipment. The rationale behind this rule is that the machines are highly sensitive and can be damaged by the smoke. Human beings are also very sensitive and can be damaged by cigarette smoke . . . A company that has demonstrated such concern for its mechanical components should have at least as much concern for its human beings.

Other lawsuits have achieved varying degrees of success, but as a general strategy, litigation is extremely limited, as it is very expensive, can last for years, and is subject to reversal upon judicial review. A specific decision, moreover, can be interpreted so narrowly as to affect only the individual litigant.

RESPONSE OF THE TOBACCO INDUSTRY TO PASSIVE SMOKING CANCER STUDIES

The popularity of legislative and other approaches to limiting passive exposure to cigarette smoke has provoked a range of responses from the tobacco industry itself. Any response at all seems remarkable, because for many years the industry has shied away from making unsolicited public comments on health issues, partly out of fear of inadvertently making statements which could be used in the enormous personal injury suits which have been filed against them (Ernster, 1986).

At present, however, the industry is divided on what public posture it should take. R. J. Reynolds has run full-page ads depicting the problem as one of "common courtesy" and "smokers' rights," rather than of health hazards. Philip Morris, on the other hand, has portrayed clean air advocates as dangerous zealots, who, in the words of its Vice-Chairman, could as easily attack "someone else's right to pray or choose a place to live. So the real issue isn't smoking versus non-smoking—it's discrimination versus tolerance." The fact that industry spokesmen are taking such an aggressive tack in public, after years of self-imposed silence, is impressive evidence of their deep concern about the success of anti-smoking and clean indoor air campaigns.

WHY PASSIVE SMOKING IS AN IMPORTANT PUBLIC HEALTH CONCERN

Passive smoking involves involuntary exposure of large numbers of people to an agent, cigarette smoke, which is well established as a cause of cancer in smokers and of other illnesses in non-smokers exposed to it. This agent contains high concentrations of known carcinogens. Therefore, even in the absence of epidemiologic evidence such exposure would be deemed potentially carcinogenic. Some epidemiologic studies, moreover, have shown lung cancer risk to be higher in women exposed to second-hand cigarette smoke. Such evidence is by no means unanimous or entirely consistent, but limitations inherent in epidemiological methods may make it impossible for us ever to be as certain about the health risks of passive smoking as we are about active smoking itself.

Many new studies of cancer risks from passive smoking are now in progress which take into account the problems encountered in earlier studies, and will undoubtedly lead to revision of the risk estimates made in those reports. It is unlikely, however, that the main conclusion (that an increased cancer risk exists) will be discarded; rather, it will probably be strengthened.

The consensus within the public health community is that it is neither necessary nor desirable to wait for "absolute proof" of causation, and that data now available justify acting on public health principles to limit, insofar as possible, public exposure to second-hand smoke. The legislative and other activities described in this paper are based upon these considerations.

If the positive reports are indeed correct, the magnitude of the increase in risk for the non-smoker is on the order of 1.3 to 3.4 times the risk in the unexposed. Few case-control studies reported so far have had the very large sample size necessary to detect risks of this magnitude with reasonable statistical power, which may be an additional reason that some studies did not confirm an effect (Weiss, 1986). Even a fairly small relative risk, however, can translate into a large number of affected persons in a population as large as the United States. Repace and Lowrey, for example, have estimated that as many as 5,000 lung cancers per year which occur in non-smokers may be attributable to passive smoking (Repace and Lowrey, 1985).

Passive smoking should therefore be of special concern to non-smoking women who are married to smokers, or who work in an environment where others are permitted to smoke. In addition, women smokers should be aware of the health risks which they may create in the non-smokers they live and work with, and particularly the children they have or may be expecting.

REFERENCES

Ayer, H.E., & Yeager, D.W. (1982). Irritants in cigarette smoke plumes. *Am J Public Health* 72:1283–1285.

Bonham, G.S., & Wilson, R.W. (1981). Children's health in families with cigarette smokers. *Am J Public Health* 71:290–293.

Brunnemann, K.D., & Hoffmann, D. (1978). Chemical studies on tobacco smoke. LIX. Analysis of volatile nitrosamines in tobacco smoke and polluted indoor environments. In E.A.Walker, L.Griciute, M.Castegnaro, R.E.Lyle, & W.Davis (Eds.) *Environmental aspects of N-nitroso compounds*. IARC Publ. No. 19 (pp. 343–356). Lyon, France: International Agency for Research on Cancer.

Butler, N.R., Goldstein, H., & Ross, E.M. (1972). Cigarette smoking in pregnancy: Its influence on birth weight and perinatal mortality. *Brit Med J* 2:127–130.

Chan, W.C., & Fung, S.C. (1982). Lung cancer in nonsmokers in Hong Kong. In *Cancer Campaign*, Vol. 6: *Cancer Epidemiology*. E. Grundmann, Ed. New York: Gustav Fischer Verlag.

Charlton, A. (1984). Children's coughs related to parental smoking. *Brit Med J* 288:1647–1649.

Comstock, G.W., Shak, F.K., Meyer, M.B., & Abbey, H. (1971). Low birth weight and neonatal mortality rate related to maternal smoking and socioeconomic status. *Am J Obstet Gynecol* 111:53–59.

Correa, P., Pickle, L.W., Fontham, E., Lin, Y., & Haenszel, W. (1983). Passive smoking and lung cancer. *Lancet* 2:595–597.

Ernster, V.L. (1986). Women, smoking, cigarette advertising and cancer. *Women and Health* 11:217–235.

Friedman, G.D., Petitti, D.B., & Bawol, R.D. (1983). Prevalence and correlates of passive smoking. *Am J Public Health* 73:401–405.

Garfinkel, L. (1981). Time trends in lung cancer mortality among nonsmokers and a note on passive smoking. *J Natl Cancer Inst* 66:1061–1066.

Garfinkel, L., Auerbach, O,. & Joubert, L. (1985) Involuntary smoking and lung cancer: A case-control study. *J Natl Cancer Inst* 75:463–469.

Goujard, J., Rumeau, C., & Schwartz, D. (1975). Smoking during pregnancy, stillbirth and abruptio placentae. *Biomedicine* 23:20–22.

Greenberg, R.A., Haley, N.J., Etzel, R.A., & Loda, F.A. (1984). Measuring the exposure of infants to tobacco smoke. Nicotine and cotinine in urine and saliva. *New Engl J Med* 310:1075–1078.

Harlap, S., & Davies, A.M. (1974). Infant admissions to hospital and maternal smoking. *Lancet* 1:529–532.

Himmelberger, D.U., Brown, B.W., & Cohen, E.N. (1978) Cigarette smoking during pregnancy and the occurrence of spontaneous abortion and congenital abnormality. *Am J Epidemiol* 108:470–479.

Hirayama, T. (1981). Non-smoking wives of heavy smokers have a higher risk of lung cancer: A study from Japan. *Brit Med J* 282:183–185.

Hoffmann, D., Haley, N.J., Adams, J.D. & Brunnemann, K.D. (1984). Tobacco sidestream smoke: Uptake by nonsmokers. *Prev Med* 13:608–618.

Jarvis, M.J., Russell, M.A.H., Feyerabend, D., Eiser, J.R., Morgan, M., Gammage, P., & Gray, E.M. (1985). Passive exposure to tobacco smoke: Saliva cotinine concentrations in a representative population sample of non-smoking schoolchildren. *Brit Med J* 291: 927–929.

Kabat, G.C., & Wynder, E.L. (1984). Lung cancer in nonsmokers. *Cancer* 53:1214–1221.

Kauffmann, F., Tessier, J-F., & Oriol, P. (1983). Adult passive smoking in the home environment: A risk factor for chronic airflow limitation. *Am J Epidemiol* 117:269–280.

Knight, A., & Breslin, A.B.X. (1985). Passive cigarette smoking and patients with asthma. *Med J Austral* 142:194–195.

Koo, L.C., Ho, J.H.-C., & Saw, D. (1983). Active and passive smoking among female lung cancer patients and controls in Hong Kong. *J Exp Clin Cancer Res* 4:367–375.

Kornegay, H.R., Kastenbaum, M.A., Mantel, N., Harris, J.E., DuMouchel, W.H., Macdonald, E.J., & Hirayama, T. (1983). Non-smoking wives of heavy smokers have a higher risk of lung cancer (letters to editor). *Brit Med J* 283:914–917.

Kullander, S., & Kallen, B. (1971). A prospective study of smoking and pregnancy. *Acta Obstet Gynecol Scand* 50:83–94.

Lebowitz, M.D., & Burrows, B. (1976). Respiratory symptoms related to smoking habits of family adults. *Chest* 69:48–50.

McIntosh, I.D. (1984). Smoking and pregnancy. II. Offspring risks. *Public Health Rev* 12:29–63.

Repace, J.L. (1984). Consistency of research data on passive smoking and lung cancer. *Lancet* 1:506.

Repace, J.L., & Lowery, A.H. (1985). A quantitative estimate of nonsmokers' lung cancer risk from passive smoking. *Environment International* 11:3–22.

Rickert, W.S., Robinson, J.C., & Collishaw, N. (1984). Yields of tar, nicotine, and carbon monoxide in the sidestream smoke from 15 brands of Canadian cigarettes. *Am J Public Health* 74:228–231.

Sandler, D.P., Everson, R.B., & Wilcox, A.J. (1985a). Passive smoking in adulthood and cancer risk. *Am J Epidemiol* 121:37–48.

Sandler, D.P., Wilcox, A.J., & Everson, R.B. (1985b). Cumulative effects of lifetime passive smoking on cancer risk. *Lancet* 1:312–314.

Schenker, M.B., Samet, J.M., & Speizer, F.E. (1983). Risk factors for childhood respiratory disease. The effect of host factors and home environmental exposures. *Am Rev Resp Dis* 128:1038–1043.

Shephard, R.J., Collins, R., & Silverman, F. (1979). Responses of exercising subjects to acute "passive" cigarette smoke exposure. *Environ Res* 19:279–291.

Stein, Z., & Kline, J. (1983). Smoking, alcohol, and reproduction. *Am J Public Health* 73:1154–1156, (editorial).

Trichopoulos, D., Kalandidi, A., Sparros, L., & MacMahon B. (1981). Lung cancer and passive smoking. *Int J Cancer 27:1–4*.

Trichopoulos, D., Kalandidi, A., & Sparros L. (1983). Lung cancer and passive smoking: Conclusion of Greek study. *Lancet* 2:678–679.

Trundle, J.I., & Skellern, G.C. (1983). Gas chromatographic determination of nicotine in human breast milk. *J Clin Hosp Pharmacol* 8:289–293.

Tsokos, C.P., Macdonald, E.J., Lee, P.N., & Hirayama, T. (1981). Non-smoking wives of heavy smokers have a higher risk of lung cancer (letters to editor). *Brit Med J* 283:1464–1466.

U.S. Department of Health, Education, and Welfare, (1979). *Smoking and Health: A Report of the Surgeon-General*. DHEW Publication No. (PHS) 79–50066. USDHEW, Public Health Service, Office on Smoking and Health, pp. 11–6 to 11–24.

U.S. Department of Health and Human Services. (1980). *The Health Consequences of Smoking For Women: A Report of the Surgeon-General*. USDHHS. Public Health Service, Office on Smoking and Health.

Ware, J.H., Dockery, D.W., Spiro, A., Speizer, F.E., & Ferris, B.G. (1984). Passive smoking, gas cooking, and respiratory health of children living in six cities. *Am Rev Resp Dis* 129:366–374.

Weber, A. (1984). Annoyance and irritation by passive smoking. *Prev Med* 13:618–625.

Weiss, S.T. (1986). Passive smoking and lung cancer. What is the risk? *Am Rev Resp Dis* 133:1–3.

Winn, D.M., & Pickle, L.W. (1986). Smokeless tobacco and cancer in women: Implications for cancer research. *Women and Health* 11:253–266.

Wu, A.H., Henderson, B.E., Pike, M.C., & Yu, M.C. (1985). Smoking and other risk factors for lung cancer in women. *J Natl Cancer Inst* 74:747–751.